Forty Years Behind the Mask

Micheal Hopkins

Shywind Creations, Micheal Hopkins
micheal@shywindcreations.com

ISBN-13: 978-1946117243
ISBN: 10: 1-946117242

DEDICATION

I want to dedicate this book to those who I have worked with over the past forty plus years, and to all those who have been in the trenches of surgery.

I also especially wish to dedicate this book to the woman who has lived through the circus that I have worked in for so many years. To my beautiful wife, Carol, who always knows what my day was like by the look on my face when I get home.

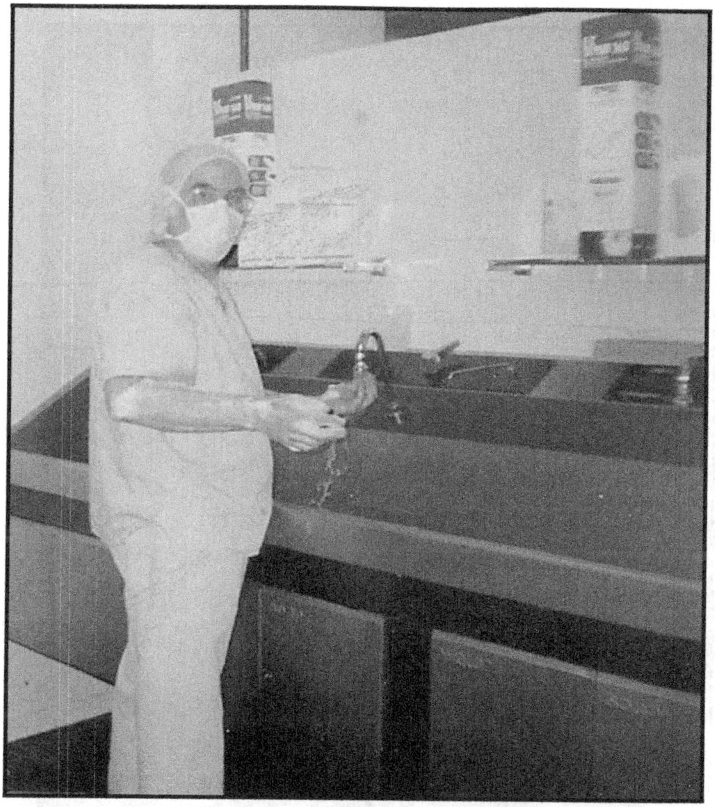

Scrubbing In

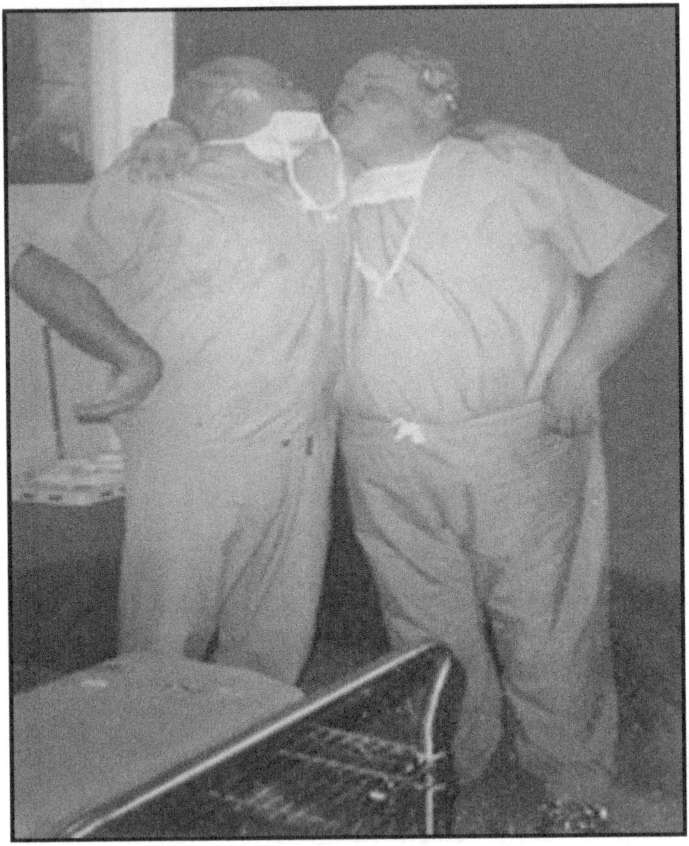

My friend Dave and I goofing around.

ACKNOWLEDGMENTS

To those who know the game of surgery, those who played by the rules, and those who didn't play by the rules, thank you for your participation in my life.

To David Morton, my dear friend and sometimes coworker, we lived these stories and experienced together both the pain and the laughter.

To Sara Dean, who kindly edited this book. Thank you for not throwing your hands in the air and demanding to know if I ever took an English Grammar Course. To be honest, I read about such a course once, but it was just too wordy.

Introduction

I guess the best way to start this book would be an introduction as to who I am and what gives me the right to tell tales out of surgery. My name is Micheal Hopkins, and I have worked in surgery for the last forty-four years. Just this admission of how long I have been in the surgical field is mind boggling to me. Imagine the human suffering that can be seen in a surgical setting over four decades. Seeing everything that can happen to the human body either by malice, accident, genetics, or fate makes me question my sanity for not being affected by it. The longer a person works in surgery or a hospital setting the thicker your skin becomes. You can stand and do your job while the patient is screaming, crying, or begging for relief. This is not a coldness by nature, it really is a defensive response to allow us to do our job. Luckily surgery patients, for the most part, are drugged and asleep. The drugged patient is often surprising and thought provoking. Do the drugs in surgery make you crazy, taking away who you really are?

Or do these drugs remove the inhibitions guarding who you really are?

But before we get into all that, we should start where every story does, at the beginning. Here's the beginning of mine…

At the tender age of nineteen I learned how to be a combat medic. Two years later I was out of the army and on my own in the big civilian world, with a great skill set. I could treat gunshot, grenade, and bayonet wounds with great skill. However, in the early seventies there was very little call for this in the everyday civilian world, so jobs were scarce to say the least. So in 1974 I joined the United States Air Force to learn a skill that I could use in the civilian world. The Air Force offered me many career choices, including computers, but I refused, figuring that computers were not going to be a big deal. They offered me air traffic control and again, I refused. I was offered crypto and language school but I declined that too. Looking back at my choices, I gave away a great career and civilian retirement in several fields. Instead I decided to train as a surgical scrub tech. I was looking forward to surgery because of the glamour, the gratitude, the feeling of personal accomplishment. What I got was long hours and lost weekends, but such are the penalties of making the wrong choice.

Many years ago, my oldest friend in the world asked me to come work at the company that employed him. I thought about it and for the second time in my life, I refused a career in computers. My friend retired at the age of sixty-two with enough money to buy a farm and travel when and where he pleased without financial worry. I am still working and he still laughs at me when we talk. I guess I have made some bad choices in my life but being a scrub tech has given me steady employment, no layoffs, and more laughs than I can count.

Over the last forty-four years working in huge facilities and one operating room hospitals, I have seen more human folly and surgical slapstick then I could ever recount. In my world of surgery there are fools, jokers, clowns, and pompous asses. They come in all shapes, sizes, genders, and ethnic backgrounds.

Some spoke English masterfully, others not so much. I met masters of their trade and bumbling fools who somehow passed medical school. But despite their differences, one thing above all else remains the same about those I have worked with - people are hilarious.

Several months ago, a longtime friend and I were discussing the weird and crazy things we have seen in surgery over the years. Dave works as a nurse anesthetist and shares my theory that surgery is a madhouse with the inmates directing the show. So, over a few drams of excellent single malt Scotch, we reminisced. We discussed the various surgeons and OR personnel from our shared assignments. Eventually we started to tell stories of the places we worked separately around the country. Here are some of those stories.

Some names and locations have been changed to protect the innocent, me.

Chapter 1

I began working in surgery for real, as in not in school, in November 1974. Working in a five hundred bed Air Force Regional Hospital afforded a new scrub tech many opportunities both professionally and comically. In this, and I believe every other hospital in the world, surgeons are envisioned as blood soaked ogres. While the idea of being an ogre was appealing to us, we were rarely blood soaked. Modern surgery has very little blood unless it's from trauma prior to surgery or a nicked artery. Regardless, the rest of the hospital personnel think we walk in pools of blood with various body parts floating merrily about. We really did nothing to fore-stall such beliefs. Sure, we would eat in the cafeteria and talk about how the above knee amputation looked so much like the prime rib we were eating, and the non-surgical crew would gather up their plates and hustle off to a table where they could look at us in horror but not hear the conversation, but was that really any reason to assume we were ogres?

My first six months as an Air Force scrub tech or surgical technologist were uneventful. Nobody lost a body part on the floor or down the linen chute. Our officer in charge, or OIC, seemed to be happy and was not making our lives miserable. Contrary to what she might think, we were not playing pranks on her to make her life miserable either.

When the OIC was on the prowl we would find ways to avenge ourselves for her annoyance. When she would do a surprise inspection of the surgical suite looking for the smallest infraction, we would put K-Y jelly mixed with methylene blue on her phone earpiece and call her from the break room. Upon answering the phone, she would have a blue slimy ear for her efforts while we had a great laugh for ours. However, pranks against our OIC really were a double-edged sword. We would have our laugh and she would then issue extra duties to the crew for after work hours. I am not sure how many times you can clean and shine the four autoclaves in our operating room, but if memory serves me right, you can do it several times a week. Now don't get me wrong, our OIC was not a complete monster, she protected us from others. Her standard reply to anyone wanting to punish one of us was, "These are my people and only I will punish my people. Now leave!" Maybe it was one of those sick love, hate, hate, love situations.

We worked hard and played hard, sometimes mixing the two together. The crew found time to do some of the stupidest pranks in the most serious way. Our senior tech was always doing something to mess with the infrastructure of the hospital. One of his favorite pranks was to take a can of Coca-Cola and place it in a vacuum delivery tube. He would then open the top and send it to another department. The soda in the can would run down the tubes into the basement center, messing up the whole system. He stopped the prank when the hospital commander ordered the finger printing of everyone in the hospital. Luckily, he always wore latex gloves when doing his pranks.

The phone system in the hospital became a great source of mischief for us as well. We would answer it in different ways just to see what laughs we could get. On one slow, lazy Friday, with all of us sitting around in the lounge waiting for the clock to send us home, the phone rang and one of the nurses picked it up. "County Morgue, You stabb'em we slab'em. Which stiff do you want?" he asked.

"Do you know who this is?" demanded the voice on the other end of the line.

"Nope, who is this?"

"I am the hospital commander!"

"Sir, do you know who this is?" the nurse asked.

"No!"

"Good!" he said and slammed the phone down into its cradle.

"I think we best get our asses out of here.

We may be having company," he said. We scattered like dead leaves in a wind storm.

I never knew if anything came of that exchange, but our OIC would sometimes give us strange looks with a small smirk after that.

The second time our lack of phone etiquette almost landed us in hot water came after we finished some cases none of us liked to do. We were doing TAB's which stands for 'Therapeutic Abortions'. This day was particularly irritating owing to the daughter of a colonel having her third procedure in thirteen months. Seems she thought it was a good form of birth control. We thought she was a little tramp. It was ten minutes before we could leave and the phone rang. One of our senior nurses answered it. "Sheppard Abortion Clinic. No fetus can beat us." She paused and then said, "I don't really care who you are. Good-bye." She slammed down the phone and left. We were all looking at her when she turned and said, "If I were you I would get the hell out of here now and don't look back!" We made rapid exits from the lounge, while calling to her, wanting to know who she had pissed off. Over her shoulder she replied,

"The deputy base commander."

Finding this out, we moved at a much more rapid, albeit quieter, pace to our lockers. I think we set records for changing and leaving. No one dared to use the main elevator, instead stairs were the preferred route of exit. The next day our OIC called us all together and told us we were expected in the office of the hospital commander in five minutes. She then smiled a genuine smile and said, "I don't know what you delinquents did but you have really pissed someone off that is very high up. I wish I could go with you to see how this plays out but I have to cancel the day's schedule."

This didn't seem like a good sign her canceling the day's schedule, which was a light one, but still. Like good little troops we went to the first floor and the office of the hospital commander. As we entered the outer office where the secretary sat we were greeted with her applause. She told us, "Head on in, they are waiting for you and may God have mercy on your black souls." Not a very encouraging prelude to our meeting.

As we entered the office we snapped to attention and saluted. The commander told us, "Be at ease. Take a slip of paper, pick up that phone, and speak what is written on the paper into it."

We each took our slip of paper, and as we read it there were snickers and suppressed laughter from the group. Each slip read the same thing: "Sheppard Abortion Clinic. No fetus can beat us." So, we each, in turn picked up the phone, read the words and then hung up. As the senior nurse who made the fateful comment took the phone she read the words in the greatest southern drawl I have ever heard. The deputy base commander was on the other end trying to find the perpetrator by the sound of the voice. It didn't work, but it was a great try on his part.

After the prerequisite chewing out from the hospital commander, and admonitions to not let something like this ever happen again, we left. Upon returning to the operating room our OIC counted heads and laughed.

"So, no one was caught, you delinquents are

lucky. Now get out of here and go have a drink or two so you can laugh at the system again." We took her advice and discussed her actions among ourselves. We decided she knew what had happened and she probably suspected who did it. We finally decided she should receive a certain status among the other OIC's for having such a successfully belligerent crew. After that we were less malicious to her and she still smirked every time something happened.

We played pranks on each other and some of them were just down right mean but no service personnel were hurt in the playing of these pranks. Well not hurt physically but we may have damaged a few psyches. Two that come to the forefront of my memory are assault against a superior officer and the creation of great mental anguish to a patient in our care. I will start with the presumed assault against a superior officer.

We had a lieutenant who was really into the title game. We knew her first name was Chris, so, when we talked to her we called her Chris and she would correct us, telling us her name was

Lieutenant, followed by her last name. I am not sure who came up with the idea for the prank but I was not involved, although I admit I did have knowledge of what was going to happen.

I was in surgery when it came down. It seems Lieutenant Last Name was walking down a back hall in surgery when an unknown person, or persons, placed a canvas linen sack over her body, cinched it up and put her on the linen cart, loaded the cart onto the elevator, and sent her down to the laundry. Needless to say, but I will say it anyway, she was rather angry when she finally returned to surgery. As I mentioned earlier, yes, I knew what was afoot but had absolutely no hand in the act. This didn't seem to matter to Chris when she entered the operating room where I was assisting in a gallbladder operation. She walked up behind me and whispered, "So you think that was funny? You think you can get away with what you did?"

I replied, "Honest to God Chris, I don't know what you are talking about. As you can see this has been my home for a while."

Chris replied, "Bullshit, Mikey boy, I know

your style." She opened the back of my scrub gown and proceeded to cut my pants and underwear off, grab the cut garments, and walk out of the room. I stood there with my scrub gown open and my bare butt hanging out for the world to see. This was embarrassing enough, but

then my circulator walked over and held my gown open for a better view. Finally satisfied with what she was viewing she walked over to the supply cabinet and retrieved an iodoform drape. This drape is golden yellow in color with a very sticky adhesive. Opening the package and walking back over she placed the sticky side down on my bare hair covered bottom and wrapped me tightly for propriety. I now had a mini skirt of surgical barrier all the way around my hips, privates, and bottom. When this task was finished my circulator commented for the first time, "There you go Hopkins, at least you are covered. I won't say you are decent simply because I don't think you have any decency in you, but that is not important." Turning and walking back to her desk, she was applauded by the other officers in the room.

I was standing there with a cold, sticky, hair pulling torture device around my lower body and she thought I had no decency. I was appalled! Well not really, but still it was embarrassing. Just when things seemed they couldn't get any worse I heard the door to the room open and the voice of my OIC ring out, "Sergeant Hopkins, I don't know what you are trying to do here but I will be happy to listen. Be in my office as soon as the case is over." And then she turned and walked from the room.

Now I am one who always follows orders and 'as soon as' means 'as soon as'. Our case ended and I removed my gown and gloves, put them in the proper receptacles, and took my instruments to the cleaning room for initial processing. As I turned around I found that a group of my coworkers had followed me and were waiting outside the door. Looking at them, it seemed my coworkers, who had once seemed so professional and compassionate, had been replaced by a giggling gaggle of rubberneckers. What they were giggling about eluded me as I checked my apparel. I was wearing a green scrub top that fell to mid-hip, a large ioban drape that covered me from waist to mid-thigh, and green surgical tennis shoes over black socks. "What the hell are you people looking at?" I asked.

"Um, Sergeant Hopkins, you seem to look

different; not strange or anything, but, well, you know, different. To be honest the skirt becomes you."

The only reply that came to my lips couldn't be said, as one would be advised to not tell the officers in the group to go 'F' themselves. After finishing up the instruments it was time to go see the OIC. Standing in front of her office door I hesitated before knocking, wondering if I should have spruced myself up some. You know, like putting on scrub pants after removing the ioban, but she did say immediately, so there I stood. Taking a deep breath, I knocked and entered. "Sergeant Hopkins reporting as ordered, ma'am." This was accompanied by the sharpest salute that could be mustered.

"Hopkins, what is it with you? Are you my special atonement for sins of my youth?"

"Ma'am, the sergeant doesn't know what to say as what you refer too is not clear. What have I done to cause you to state this? I have never done anything to merit coming to your office before."

"I know about you. It's true you never are involved in the pranks, but you have a way of egging people on with questions about what if someone did this or that. Your type has been in the military since the beginning of time. Up to now it's been humorous to watch the game but today is different. You crossed the line when you sent the lieutenant down to the laundry."

I started to protest when she told me to be silent and listen. "The deputy hospital commander was doing an inspection in the laundry when your special package arrived. He was not amused to find one of his officers in a laundry bag, and even less amused when she told him she fell into the bag by accident and that's how she found her way to the laundry."

My respect for Chris jumped a thousand percent with this information and I decided it was time to include her on the prank team.

"Now you listen and you listen well Hopkins, if you are involved or if I even think you are involved in any more of these pranks that involve assaulting my officers, I will turn you over to the deputy hospital commander so fast your head will spin! Do I make myself clear?"

What response is there to such a fine option as that other than, "Yes, ma'am." I was then dismissed and told that I was out of uniform for duty and it would be best if I got into uniform post haste.

Did I mention that Ioban is very sticky and loves to stay where its placed until it is pulled off? Usually the areas we place this barrier on are shaved and prepped; unfortunately, I was neither. As I was removing it, loudly exclaiming joy with each pull, there was a knock on the locker room door. A voice on the other side asked if I needed any assistance in removing the Ioban. My response was an emphatic, "NO, Lieutenant Chris, I do not need your help." There was laughter on the other side, followed by silence.

Keeping my word to not assault officers with pranks proved quite easy, since there were bigger fish to fry. My senior sergeant was having difficulty with his private parts. Basically, he

suffered with phimosis, a condition in which the foreskin on the penis will not retract over the glans. It is uncomfortable at best and painful as hell at worst. My sergeant Cliff, was suffering the worst. He complained that the condition destroyed his love life. If the foreskin did roll back it might tear or worse, get trapped behind the glans. The remedy for this condition is a circumcision and consequently Cliff was scheduled for one that Friday. That gave us three days to ponder what we could do to make his surgical experience memorable. It was Chris of the laundry bag who came up with the perfect gag.

Friday rolled around and everything was in place. The surgeon knew his lines, anesthesia had his ducks in a row and the rest of the staff in the room were ready. Earlier during the week Chris had lunch with Cliff's wife and filled her in on what was going to happen. She was one hundred percent on board with us. (She was delightfully twisted.)

I was the lead scrub tech during the circumcision since, as Cliff put it, “Even you can’t screw up a circ now can you, Hopkins?” Poor Cliff if he only knew. The case started like all cases with everyone ready for their part in the procedure. Anesthesia gave Cliff a spinal because he didn’t want to go to sleep for the procedure. Everything was ready, so very ready. The urologist was in fine humor and worked very quickly performing the operation and suturing everything in place. He looked at me and nodded. I looked at Chris and nodded. She indicated she was ready and the games began.

The surgeon was making a show of using his scalpel to do the procedure while describing to Cliff what he was doing. This was all window dressing, we were done with the surgery and now it was time for the prank. As the surgeon was going through the motions of cutting he let out a huge sneeze and jerked his whole body. He looked down and said in a very loud voice, “Oh Shit!”

This was my cue and I responded with, “Doc, can you reattach that?”

He looked at me and said, "We have to put this on ice immediately." He turned to Chris, handing her a kidney basin with gauze over the top. "Get this on ice immediately, Chris." Taking the basin Chris started for the door.

Cliff was alert and asked, "What is going on? What do you need ice for? Answer me!"

Chris was hurrying from the room when she tripped and the kidney basin flew into the air, turning over and spilling the contents into free flight. What Cliff saw was something long and brown and bloody tumbling in open space. He let out a yell, "What the hell? Is that what I think it is? Tell me!" The anesthetist now gave Cliff a bolus of drugs to put him to sleep.

We all had a great laugh over Cliffs reaction, complimenting Chris on her acting and clumsiness. She bowed, picked up the polish sausage from the floor, and deposited it in the trash while we put the special dressing on Cliff.

We sent our patient to the recovery room where his wife was waiting and asking how it went. We told her it had been a success so far but when Cliff woke up would be the true answer. We were all sitting in the recovery room as we waited for him to wake up. Eventually Cliff awoke and was very groggy. This was his wife's cue to sob quietly and pat his hand saying, "It's okay honey, it's okay, we can deal with it."

Cliff's eyes snapped wide open and he thrusts his hands down into his groin. He frantically felt around and screams, "Where is it? What have the bastards done with it?" By this time, we couldn't control ourselves and we all started to laugh his wife included. Cliff now wide awake screamed, "You white bastards what have you done to me?" His wife took his hands and moved them down to where we had taped his penis to the inside of his thigh and reassured him, "It's okay honey, we just played a joke on you. Everything is just fine."

Cliff finally realized he had been pranked and started to laugh, then stopped looked at all of us and warned, "Of course you know this means war. I will get everyone of you somehow, someday." That however, is another story and not mine to tell.

Pranking was not the only source of humor or shock in our surgical suite. We had doctors who gave us no end of entertainment. I can distinctly remember three happenings that defy being buried in forgotten memory. The first is probably the strangest, or so it was to me.

I had been assigned to the hospital right out of tech school, which meant I received no money for travel since the school was one half mile from the hospital.

Shortly after my assignment as permanent party personnel, and after my orientation to the surgical suite, I was put into the regular rotation for cases. Now on the outside this sounds straight forward but it was anything but. Case in point - no one liked to work in neuro, well, actually, no one liked to work with this one neuro surgeon. It had nothing to do with the service nor his personality, he was a very pleasant human being. However, he had some eccentric habits that some people found hard to deal with and so assignment to his room was done by the random drawing of names.

Shortly after I entered the rotation for all

rooms an amazing situation arose. It seemed that every time there was a day with this surgeon my name was drawn as the tech. Now random means random, but with my luck at being drawn weekly I should have purchased lottery tickets! I became a little suspicious that maybe 'random' had some outside influence when the drawing occurred. After the third time of being drawn for neuro little warning bells started to ring in my head. So, that day after surgery I sneaked into the NCOIC's office and pulled my name from the box. The next week a miracle occurred - my name was drawn yet again!

It seemed strange to me, but I figured what the hell, maybe he just noticed my name was missing and replaced it. Once again I sneaked into the NCOIC's office and searched for the offending name chit. Amazingly my chit was not in there. Hmm, what could this mean? Well, it meant I was going to be in the neuro room every week so it would be smart to just make the best of it.

I learned my neuro surgeon knew very important people. In conversation during a routine spinal fusion it was revealed to me that my surgeon discussed cases with Sir Winston Churchill on a routine basis. Now why was this of any importance you might ask? Well, this time frame was in the early seventies and Churchill had passed in 1965. So, my mental question was, was he psychic or psychotic? The answer eluded me.

He had other habits that took some getting used to as well. Such as stopping in the middle of an open skull case and telling me it was time for coffee and a smoke. At which point he removed his gown and gloves and I mine. The circulator would get a cup of coffee for anesthesia and one for herself. Everyone copes as best they can, one would assume. I would follow the doctor to the break room where he would bum a cigarette from me, pour us both a cup of coffee and grab the newspaper to look through the obituaries to see if anyone he knew had passed in the night. During one of these breaks he started to talk about how the night before he had discussed that day's case with Sir Winston. Taken by surprise I asked, "Sir Winston?"

"Yes, Sir Winston Churchill. We have discussed my cases for several years now. He really makes me aware of what needs to be done." Finishing his coffee, he got up and we returned to surgery and finished the case. Not being sure of my memory, I looked up Sir Winston Churchill and saw he had passed a few years earlier. This left me wondering if I should be around this doctor when he had sharp objects in his hand. Over the next few months he showed no signs of attacking me with a scalpel or a drill so I was far less nervous around him.

We were in a skull case being done under local anesthesia so that the patient could interact with the surgeon about what they saw smelled, tasted, heard, or felt. As we were working on the brain the patient let out a loud, "OUCH!" This prompted the surgeon to look at the patient and ask, "What did that feel like?" The patient responded, "It hurt." My surgeon just rolled his eyes and he set back to work. A few minutes later the patient let out another loud, "OUCH!" This prompted the surgeon to stop work and look the patient directly in the eyes.

He informed the patient there was no pain and the patient replied, "Yes, there is. I feel it."

The man who discussed cases with Sir Winston Churchill, grabbed the patients nose, informing him that, "The pain you feel does not hurt so please be quiet." Strangely enough the patient made no further outburst during the procedure. Did he feel pain or not is of no consequence, what matters is the surgeon's explanation.

Curiosity finally forced me to ask the doctor if he discussed his cases with Sir Winston Churchill or if he was just pulling my leg? The doctor looked at me with a hurt expression on his face and said, "I talk to Winston every night about the next day's surgeries. He gives me insight into the case which is unique, and I find the input to be very useful." Having explained this, he turned back to his newspaper and read the obituaries yet again. It was not until many months later the others in the unit let me in on the secret - Sir Winston Churchill was the doctor's English bulldog. Somehow I just didn't feel any better knowing about his dog.

I had the privilege of working with a very fine urologist; this man was a surgeon that wasted no time. Besides being fast, he had the misfortune to also be very good. This surgeon was blessed with a sense of humor and a very quick wit. During a routine case to fix a ureter damaged during a gynecological case performed a couple days earlier, his quick wit manifested itself. Out of the corner of his eye he glimpsed something fluttering in the room. "Nurse, is that a butterfly over in the corner?" This, of course brought all our attention to the corner, and sure enough there was a very lovely butterfly setting on a cabinet. Our surgeon turned from the patient after telling us to not do anything stupid and walked over to the cabinet. He removed his gloves and gentle as could be, he coaxed the butterfly into his hands. Taking it over to the circulator he told her, "Get a large container cleaned with no formaldehyde and poke holes in the lid. Make out a pathology sheet and write the following: Found in patient's abdomen. What do you make of it? Sign my name and send it down to pathology stat."

With the order given and information entered

the specimen was sent to the pathologist. Having nothing better to do we returned to the case having a good chuckle about how the pathologist must be reacting to our specimen. Surprisingly enough we didn't have to wait very long to find out. The phone in the room rang. Our circulator answered the phone and put it on speaker for all to hear. "Hello, is this Doctor Bull?"

Our doctor replied, "Yes, this is he. How may I help you?"

"This is Doctor Johnson in pathology and I have your specimen before me."

"Oh yes, the specimen, well doctor what do you make of it?"

"Analysis of the specimen has shown that your patient is extremely nervous and would benefit from a nerve calming agent."

"Thank you, Doctor Johnson. I appreciate your prompt attention to this request."

"No problem. I regret to inform you that we lost the specimen so we can't do a permanent on it. Unfortunately, someone left the window open and it flew out to inspect the flowers."

"No, that's quite all right. Thank you for your input. Good-bye."

"Thank you for your interesting specimen. Good-bye."

We all had another good chuckle over the butterfly when our surgeon voiced the opinion, "You know I think I will go down to path after surgery and meet this Doctor Johnson, maybe buy him a drink. He has a sense of humor. I like that."

This same surgeon who would send butterflies to pathology had a dark side too. Nothing would be tolerated that interfered with surgery. Nothing, in his case, meant nothing. We were progressing nicely during a nephrectomy on an elderly retired service member. The case was more than half done when the OIC opened the door to our room and called to the doctor, "Doctor, maintenance is going to be shutting down the electrical power to this room in ten minutes so they can work on an x-ray machine." There was complete silence in the room as we all backed away from the surgeon. We feared an explosion and wanted to be out of the blast zone.

Turning to the OIC, our surgeon very calmly stated, "I am sorry Major, I don't think I heard you correctly; probably the acoustics in the room. I will come over there and if you could repeat what you said I will be obliged." With that he turned and reached onto my mayo stand, then walked over to the OIC. "Now what were you saying about ten minutes, Major?"

Our OIC repeated what she had said earlier verbatim. When she was done, the surgeon reached up, closed a penetrating towel clip to the front of the OIC's scrubs and growled, "Now if you bring your ass over here with me, Major, I will explain why you are wrong with your message and your time." Holding the towel clip firmly he led her to the patient. "Now, if you look down here you will see that I will not be able to do what you are telling me must be done in ten minutes. I will need another three quarters of an hour to finish this case. You will notice that I am removing this man's kidney and I need lights, cautery, and anesthesia to complete what I am doing. So, you will now go out and tell maintenance to cool their heels until I am done. Do I make myself clear, Major?"

The OIC shook her head to the affirmative and croaked, "Yes, Doctor, I will take care of it right away." The doctor removed the towel clip and motioned her from the room. As she was shoving the door open she turned and said in her best commanding voice, "I will naturally tell the hospital commander of your actions."

The doctor threw the towel clamp at her, just missing her head and stated, "As I will also be telling him of your actions today, ma'am"

She scurried from the room and I changed the doctor's gloves. I then said, "You don't seem to be worried about the hospital CO taking her side."

"No, I am not worried. The CO is a surgeon

and we golf together. Nothing will come of this. And nothing did come of it.

Chapter 2

I didn't make the military a career because there was only so much regimented living I could take. Being married also had weight in my decision to not make the military a career. My lovely wife is a free spirit and does not take hassle from anyone very well. She would throw ice water on the hinges of Hell just to let the devil know she was unhappy with him, and he would take notice and back off. That is my wife and I am the luckiest man in the world.

My first civilian job as a surgical scrub tech was in Butte Montana, of all places, at The Sisters of Charity Hospital. The name sounds good but trust me, the sisters only had charity for themselves; their employees, not so much. In the military, I was making six hundred dollars a month with separate rations and housing. My pay at The Sisters figured out to one dollar and eighty-six cents an hour, with a bonus of twenty-five cents for each hour I was on call. Or as most places call it, 'stand-by pay'. All in all, I was making half of what I made in the service but I would be paid time and one half for each hour I worked on callback. I also received time and one half for any time over forty hours in a work week. And did I forget to mention I had the benefit of a union? I was required to join Teamsters Local Number Two as a requirement to work for The Sisters. After an initiation fee that cost close to half a week's pay I was welcomed as a fellow Teamster. This allowed me to give four dollars a week in union dues for the privilege of carrying the card. For some strange reason, I sort of missed the military.

The Sister's Hospital was not modern by any stretch of the imagination. There were windows facing the outside world in two of the four surgical suites. This happened because there was a need to expand surgical rooms and the cheapest solution was to divide the medical library in half and make two rooms from it. So, that is what the sisters did and consequently we had a fourth-floor window to the world.

Being a full-service hospital we had all the usual specialties to offer the community with orthopedics being the big money maker. Being the biggest money maker has it perks and ortho always had room three, one of the rooms with a view. Being a male and standing a bit over six feet tall sealed my fate with the sisters was an orthopedic tech from the start of my employment. This did not mean I worked with the ortho doctors every day they were in the hospital, it meant I was called in, regardless of who was on call to do ortho cases. However, I only received stand-by pay of twenty-five cents an hour on my call nights. The other nights I was expected to respond and that was that.

More about that later, but right now I will share the reason room three was the room the orthopedic doctors wanted. Across the street was a nice, neat three-story building that belonged to the Montana School of Mines and was used for female students. The windows in our surgery had an unobstructed view onto the roof and fenced in backyard of the building. During the late spring, the young ladies started to work on their suntans by laying out on the roof or on blankets in the back-yard. Some of the ladies wanted more of a tan than the others and consequently wore less while tanning.

The show would draw the surgeons to the windows like moths to a flame. Surgery would be delayed until either the doctors saw enough or one of the sisters would scurry into the room and admonish them for the weakness of the flesh. I never found voyeurism to be an enjoyable hobby and never went to the window. I am not purer than others, I just have different things that excite me. This went on for several years until the sisters decided to put an end to it. One Monday morning we came in for an orthopedic case and found the sisters had the maintenance department brick in the lower half of the windows so that a tall man would not be able to see anything but the sky. To me it was hilarious, to the orthopods it was an act of war at best and a heinous crime against humanity and men at the worst. Strangely, the sisters didn't seem to care how much the doctors complained and eventually the situation quieted down with just the occasional complaint.

Every morning the sisters would ring a bell

and all the surgical crew stood in the door ways and prayed as the sisters walked by chanting a prayer. We then would return to our duties, better for the delay.

Christmas was a special time in the hospital and on Christmas Eve the sisters would have an assembly in the conference room; attendance was mandatory. Even those of us who were not Catholics attended, as it was considered good for our souls and continued employment. So, I would attend and listen to an hour of prayer in Latin and some hymns. Then the sisters would admonish us with stories of the starving in the world and how we, who had so much, were obligated to help those who had so little. This was followed by a collection plate carried down the rows by a stern faced sister who would comment on the small amount of a donation and praise the larger ones. It was a 'damned if you, do damned if you don't' situation. Ten dollars elicited no comments, good or bad, and so that is what the underpaid tech would donate.

The high point of my time with The Sisters was the strike. The teamsters wanted more money for their members and consequently that equated to more money for the union as well. Contract time came and went with no satisfaction for the union or its members. We then voted to strike. When teamsters strike, it means no trucks will cross the picket lines. We figured the hospital would capitulate in short order, but instead nuns from all over the state would drive up in cars and pickups loaded with supplies for the hospital and cross the picket lines. Not even the nastiest union member would mess with a nun.

One night the union tough guys built a blockade that stopped the nuns in their tracks and the strike then continued as a strike should with one group against another with no common ground. We were on strike for three months when both sides decided it was enough and the hospital made an offer, which the union counter-offered. The hospital accepted the counter-offer and with a great deal of backslapping and hugs we went back to work. When it was all said and done my union dues went up eight cents an hour and my pay went up six cents an hour. I felt very relieved that I only lost two cents an hour over what I was making before the strike.

Time passed, which is a good thing one would suppose, however when time passes, situations change. I was tired of working for peanuts with The Sisters of Charity. So just like the Beverly Hillbillies, I loaded up the truck and headed for California to seek a more equitable wage. In Northern California I found a small county hospital that paid a staggering sum of seven dollars and eighty-three cents an hour to start. This was almost four times what I made with The Sisters of Charity! The best part - there were no union dues, no enforced morning prayers, and no nuns looking at me like I was the son of Satan.

My first day on the job I met the doctor who would make me very happy that I came to this area. Doctor David was more twisted than a pretzel. He loved practical jokes and messing with the administration on a routine basis. Doctor David was not a surgeon, but a general practitioner. In this area of Northern California, it was not uncommon for a GP to do surgery. We had a pair of fine general surgeons who also did vascular and thoracic surgery and a pair of good orthopods. But David was different, he would do most surgeries and do them very well. David would do C-sections, gall bladders, hernias, bowel resections with a general surgeon assistant, and the occasional aneurysm repair if needed. Yes, Doctor David was an interesting human being. When we first met I was gowning and gloving him and gave him my normal greeting to a doctor the first time we meet, "How would you like to be addressed?"

His response made my day.

"You can call me anything you like if its civil. I would prefer David and I know that there will be times you will want to call me asshole, but please do that under your breath."

So David and I started our professional relationship on an up note. Our first case was a bowel exploration, basically there was something wrong and we were not sure what it was. This is the reason we do exploratory procedures, which is basically a fishing or hunting trip in the body. His assistant was one of the general surgeons but in the middle of the case he was called away for an emergency trauma case involving the spleen. That left David and myself. He would search on one side and tell me to check the other. He finally found a section of dead bowel and we repaired it. I couldn't do anastomosis but he could, and did, and it was a pleasure to watch. Thus, ended our first day, and probably our last normal day, together.

Approximately two months after our initial case together Doctor David called from the emergency room to our surgical desk, and stated that there was an inbound ambulance carrying a patient with a dissecting abdominal aortic aneurysm. There was no further information but we jumped at the warning and setup a room for the coming emergency. You have no time to play games when such an emergency comes in; it is life or death with no time to play, no time to delay. We opened the room for the emergency packs, instruments, sutures, and all the other necessary supplies needed to do the case. Time passed and it was now a half hour and no patient. When it reached an hour we grew concerned. Finally, the circulator called the ER to ask about the patient. What she was told made her turn beet red and she slammed the receiver down on the phone screaming, "That rotten sucker! It was a joke! He called to prank us with a bogus case! There is no patient, no emergency, nothing!"

Needless to say, we were pissed. Not just pissed but demanding revenge! As we cleaned up and threw out several thousand dollars worth of now wasted supplies, we plotted and planned. Our decision was made and we just had to wait for the chips to fall into place. Two weeks after the Triple A incident I was on call and received a call from Doctor David. He had a patient with failure to progress and wanted to do a C-section in a half hour. He called me first because I needed to get the room opened and equipment and supplies available or opened. My response was short and to the point, "I am so sorry Doc, but I will not fall for another of your practical jokes. I will not waste more hospital money on false overtime or wasted supplies to give you a laugh. Good-bye." I hung up and waited for the call back.

The phone rang and I answered and listened to Doctor David scream, "This isn't a practical joke, its real! Now get your ass down to the hospital. I am ordering you to…" At that point I hung up and went back to bed. The rest of the crew responded the same way I did, including the director of surgery. The next day we heard that the doctor shipped the patient to a neighboring hospital for the procedure and she delivered in the ambulance. We were met at the door of surgery by the hospital administrator. He had been awakened by a very irate Doctor David and wanted some explanations and a good reason not to fire us all. We all sat down in the recovery room and told the story of the Triple A prank. We then told him that one very good reason that he couldn't fire us was that no one would be there to do surgery, thereby costing the hospital thousands of dollars a day. Having no knowledge of the Triple A prank, the administrator asked for a dollar figure on the wasted money and overtime of the crew for waiting. We gave him the information and he said, "I will be talking to you again very soon, but don't get too comfortable in your jobs just yet."

A couple hours later the administrator and Doctor David returned to the operating rooms. Doctor David apologized for the prank, promising to never do something like that again.

We didn't' really believe him, but we decided to let bygones be bygones.

The administrator then told us of Doctor David's generosity. "Doctor David has decided he should reimburse the hospital for lost money due to an unfortunate practical joke, and he will be buying lunch for the OR crew for the next week." True to his word there were no more practical jokes and for the most part that was a good thing, although boring on occasion.

Another member of the staff at this hospital was a very competent and pleasant orthopedic surgeon, I will call him George. George was a big man and for the most part a very happy-go-lucky individual. His only real fault was a belief in the powers that be, being infallible, and always making the correct decision. This belief caused many embarrassing and hilarious, situations over the years. One instance sticks out in my mind.

We, the surgery crew, had a long running battle with the human resources department of our hospital. The person in charge would do salary comparisons to give the information to the board when it came time to determine raises for the operating room staff. The basic report she sent to the board of directors started out with the same standard phrase: "It is the considered opinion of the staff in human resources that the following is a fair and honest representation of wages paid in hospitals of similar size and services as our facility." Now that is really official sounding, making it sound like the report is a consensus of opinion from human resources specialists, but there were a few problems with that. Problem number one - there was exactly one employee in human resources. Problem number two her previous position was dietary aide. She learned on the job and from reading books. Every year the board would read her recommendations and act accordingly awarding those of us in surgery with raises ranging from a quarter to fifty cents. Every year she would receive a bonus for keeping hospital expenses in HR down. And every year George would tell us how lucky we were to receive a raise.

We finally decided to act on our own behalf, run our own survey, and compare our wages to hospitals that did the same cases and caseloads as us. Our director sat down one day and called all her friends in various operating rooms around the state and compiled a spread sheet of cases done, types of cases, average cases per month, per year, and callback procedures. She then entered the average wages paid to the staff and the high and low pay scales. A few weeks later the board received the numbers from the "staff" of the human resources department and shortly after they received our numbers and documentation.

It was during this time that George told me during a surgical case that he felt we were over paid for what we did, as anyone could do our job. He explained to me and the second scrub in the room that, "We were like the people in the tool crib of a manufacturing company, we handed out the tools and took them back with no real knowledge about the use or purpose of them."

His partner Rick told him, "George I would not make statements like that to this group."

To which George responded, "Well it's true. I looked at the papers from human resources and I really think the crew should be happy with what they get."

I looked at the second scrub and she nodded, I then looked at the nurse, who also nodded. Moving back from the operating field I took off my gloves walked up behind George, and dropped his pants to the floor. George just stood there, shocked, as his partner said, "I warned you, George."

After dropping his pants, I removed my gown and walked from the room, followed by the nurse and the second scrub. The nurse turned to the silent room and explained, "If we are so worthless and easy to replace I would suggest you start now. Until there is an apology for such insulting language from you, 'DOCTOR', we will be in the lounge having coffee and a smoke."

Our director was in the lounge when we walked in and she asked, "Is the case over already?"

We explained what transpired and she doubled over with laughter, wishing she could have seen it. A few minutes later George walked in and apologized. The director informed him that that was not enough and he was expected to push for our numbers at the board meeting that night. George understood the unspoken part of that statement. Our director ran surgery and the administrator didn't mess with her, neither did the board. If she said "NO" it meant no, and it would not be changed by anyone. We received our first real raise in four years, bringing us up to the mid-range pay of hospitals we compared with in the survey. There was no bonus for the head of HR that year or any year after, and when she finally retired there was no fanfare or big hospital outflow of appreciation for her services.

I didn't relate this to show how powerful or mean we were, I want the reader to know that in bygone years employees could get things done. Sometimes the means were bizarre or rude, but we solved problems ourselves for the most part. Today we have unions that are in bed with the hospitals, we have HR departments who look only at some national average, or whatever policy is in vogue at some ivory tower institution.

The hospital I have been writing about was a treasure trove of weird creatures. There was a general surgeon who was also one of the three surgeons doing vascular surgery. I scrubbed a number of Triple A's with this man and he was good. I will call him Steve, because that is a nice name, and he for the most part, was a nice man. He had a situation at home which affected the way he ran his practice. Steve's wife was a member of the La Leche League, which means she was big into breast feeding her children. That would be fine, except in this case the children were five and seven. Steve was not allowed to touch the milk machines at home, while his children had daily free use of them. To make up for this, I believe he gave everyone who came into his office a breast exam. You came in for a hernia, you got a breast exam; you came in for varicose veins, you got a breast exam. Any exam included a breast exam regardless of the reason for the visit. Poor Steve was forced to give extra service to his patients because of his wife's beliefs.

We were called into do an emergency C-section one evening and the only other surgeon available to help in the C-section was Steve. He scrubbed in with us and we began to do our case. Not far into the procedure we heard a moan and thought that maybe the anesthesia provider was keeping the patient too light. We soon realized it was Steve, he was as pale as a ghost! He was mumbling, "Blood, so much blood, oh God, the blood!" He then staggered away from our table, bounced off the wall and wobbled out the door. He grabbed a hook for holding lab coats and proceeded to pull it off the wall as he fell in a dead faint. One of the assisting OB nurses ran out and helped him to the lounge where he could lie down. She returned laughing, and told us that Steve just couldn't take the sight of all the blood and fluid from the operation, and it made him sick. We all laughed about it and sometime the next week a plaque was put on the wall. The plaque featured a bent lab coat hook brass piece engraved with the words, "Doctor Steve's Memorial C-Section Hook". He never lived it down and we never missed the opportunity to moan, "The blood! All the blood! Ohhhhhhhh!"

Another interesting employee at the hospital was a nurse who worked in intensive care, who loved to make cakes for parties and put shaving cream somewhere in the frosting. She made great cakes but no one would eat the frosting, not even on a bet. Rumor had it that she had baked and decorated the wedding cake for her daughter's wedding and decorated the top tier with shaving cream while the rest was a delicious cream frosting.

When I started at the hospital there was an administrator who had three secretaries to keep people from getting in to see him. He told the nurses at a meeting that we were damned lucky to have a job, as replacements for us were, in his opinion a dime a dozen. So, we needed to shut up and do our job. The next day he was presented with one hundred forty-seven dimes and told to go buy a few dozen nurses because we were now tendering our resignations. He blustered and the board panicked. The administrator was terminated and replaced in a very short period of time. His secretaries were fired or reassigned and the new administrator apologized for his predecessor's actions.

One last instance of the strangeness of the surgeons at this hospital must be told. I worked with the gynecological surgeons routinely. Henry was a surgeon in the field of gynecology.

Maynard was the anesthesiologist and they absolutely hated each other. I have no idea why and really it was more fun to watch the interactions then try to figure out the reasons for the feud. Henry was a sweater, and if the temperature in the room went much above sixty-two degrees he dripped sweat. Maynard really didn't care what the room temperature was and for the most part he left it alone. Oh, did I fail to mention the temperature control was next to the anesthesia machine and Maynard had control of the settings?

As I said for the most part he would set the temperature where we requested. When Henry was in the room all bets were off and the temperature would slowly raise into the mid to upper eighties. All the techs knew that when this game started it was best to just shut up and endure the case until it was done. We would then go change our soaked scrubs and tell Maynard it was not fun to which he usually replied, "Tough."

The incidence I am going to share happened during the last case of the day, an abdominal hysterectomy with Henry and his office partner Thomas. Thomas was not a bad sort, and was really a pleasant man to be around, but he was not the world's greatest surgeon. So, he would generally take the place of a second scrub tech holding retractors and cutting sutures. When they worked together it was like a vacation for me.

In this case Maynard and Henry were on edge with each other and the rest of us were going to suffer for their moods. We were about thirty minutes into the case and it was progressing well, when the temperature in the room hit eighty and continued to climb. Henry was sweating like a glass of ice tea on a summer day, you know, covered in beads of water. As Henry was leaning into get a better look at the uterus, his glasses slipped off his nose and plummeted into the open wound. We all winced and waited for the explosion, which did not come. Henry just reached in to the wound and retrieved his glasses, then handed them to me. I washed them in a basin of sterile water I kept on the field for instruments that were bloody. I dried the glasses and replaced them on his face. I changed his gloves and my own.

The nurse replaced my basin with a fresh, non-contaminated one. Henry looked at Maynard and said, “Give her an antibiotic.”

The case continued with nothing being said about temperature or diving eyeglasses. We removed the uterus, closed the vaginal cuff, and started the process of closing the wound. I was beginning to relax when I heard Thomas mutter, “Ah hell, not again.” I looked up just in time to see Henry retrieve his glasses a second time, and hand them to me for cleaning. Judging from the look on his sweat drenched face, there were going to be words… and there were.

Henry turned to the head of the table and yelled, “Maynard you’re a worthless son of a bitch! Turn the heat down in the room now!”

Maynard looked up from his machine and very slowly, very deliberately, gave Henry the finger. Which did not make the situation any better.

Having finished cleaning the glasses again I handed them to Henry and asked, “Do you want me to get the nurse to tape them to your forehead?"

Henry looked at me without saying a word, as he reached onto the back table and grabbed the skin stapler. I watched him, wondering what he intended to do with it. I didn't have to wait to find out. He grabbed his glasses with one hand and proceeded to staple the glasses to the bridge of his nose. Seeing this made my stomach feel strange and all my body parts exhibited that strange tingle you get when something spooky happens. I quietly said, "That has to hurt more than a piece of tape would."

Henry looked at me and very softly replied, "Hopkins, aren't you just brilliant. Yes, it hurts, you stupid son of a bitch. What would you think if I put a staple in the bridge of your damned nose?"

I replied with Irish formality, "What would I think, sir? Why, I would be deciding which of your fingers to break first if you ever tried something that stupid."

Maynard looked sick to his stomach as he viewed the staple in Henry's nose. He reached up and turned the temperature in the room down to sixty degrees. Not another word was spoken in the room as we closed the patient. At the case's end Henry grabbed a hemostat and ripped the staple from the bridge of his nose before leaving the room.

Thomas looked at me and asked, "You were joking with your response to Henry weren't you? You sounded so polite and formal and all, but it was a joke, right?"

My response was, "No sir, I was not joking I meant exactly what I said; every word of it."

Thomas was looking confused when Maynard spoke up, "Tom, I have worked with Hopkins for several years and have learned to watch his eyes for clues to his moods and I saw nothing joking in his eyes when he spoke."

The next day it was business as usual with Henry. Not a word was said about the day before; that was his way.

I was going to end tales of this hospital experience here, but writing about the case with Henry and Thomas reminded me of my first meeting with Thomas. He was introduced to the crew by Henry, who said, "This is Thomas and he is my partner and friend, he is board certified and will be doing cases here."

Great introduction; very reassuring to say the least. Our first case together was a laparoscopic tubal ligation. Not as fancy or advanced compared to today's standards. It was still considered cutting edge as we were using staples to do the tubal ligation instead of burning the tubes or ligating with suture and cutting them. The staples were to replace suture and make removal of the tube easier. Our case started and Thomas was preparing to make his incision when he asked me, "Are you familiar with this procedure?"

I told him, "Yes, sir, I am and will not mess up."

He laughed and told me, "That is the least of my worries." I mentally scratched my head.

After making his incision he asked for the port and trocar. I handed him two piercing towel clips first and he looked at me as if to say, "Why would I need these?" Figuring he was messing with me, I reached over and placed them on either side of the incision, and then handed him the veress needle and syringe with saline for testing to see if he was in the abdomen. He inserted the needle and I placed the syringe on top and injected the saline. We were in, so we connected the carbon dioxide tubing to the needle and inflated the abdomen with the gas to give the belly wall separation from the abdominal contents. When we had the proper pressure of gas he pulled out the veress needle and took the port and trocar. He inserted it and we had a gas return, so we knew we were in the belly. He took the trocar out and placed the scope with the camera attached into the port and we saw that no bowel was injured, so we were golden. After the traditional look around, we placed the other two ports. After assuring ourselves that the ports were positioned properly and there were no insults to the bowel anywhere, I handed the doctor a grasper to manipulate the fallopian tubes so we could get them positioned for stapling. When he was satisfied with his grasper positioning I took the camera and handed him the stapler.

He looked at me and asked, "Where is the kleppinger so I can burn these?"

"The case was scheduled as a stapling and I don't have the kleppinger available to burn the tubes."

Thomas asked me, "What brilliant person scheduled this case with the stapler?"

"It was your office, so I would assume it was your secretary."

Thomas laughed. "No, it's my partner being difficult."

Feeling it best to drop the conversation I asked, "Would you prefer I get the kleppinger forceps and generator?"

He just shook his head and said, "We'll just do this with the stapler and get it done."

I handed the stapler to him again and he looked at it like it was an alien artifact found on another planet. After a few seconds he asked, "Have you used this with other surgeons?"

I told him I had, and that the device was simple to use and pretty much fool proof. He laughed when I said this and said something to the effect of, "They may be pretty fool proof but nature builds more enterprising fools each year."

I chuckled until I realized that he was telling me he was not familiar with this device. I started to have that sneaking tingling feeling that I was going to be doing something beyond my license again. Sure enough, Thomas handed the stapler back to me and said, "Well I guess this is as good a time as any to learn to use this device; please demonstrate its use."

I tried to explain, "Doctor I can tell you how it works, I can demonstrate on a sponge how it works, or I can talk you through how it works, but I am not supposed to do it on a patient."

Thomas nodded. "That's nice, now show me how this works on the left fallopian tube, please." To emphasize his instructions, he pulled the tube taut. I hesitated and he said, "I am the doctor and you are the tech. I am instructing you to do something which puts you under the authority of my license."

I was thinking, *You are instructing me to do something that you don't know how to do and I, unfortunately, do know how to do.* Realizing that this was really a no-win situation for me, I used the stapler, explaining as I went what I did and why I did it and what to do next. We removed the first tube and after reloading the device I handed it to him, but he shook his head and said, "You still have one more tube to demonstrate on and I am getting tired of this case."

So, with no other recourse, I demonstrated on the remaining tube and we finished the case. I looked at him and said, "So I guess this tech had best have the kleppinger and its generator available for all your tubal ligation cases."

Thomas smiled and put his hand on my shoulder. "That would probably be best, unless you like using the stapler." The kleppinger was always in the room and setup after that day when he was doing a tubal ligation.

The hospital started to grow and they replaced management and administrators.

Sometimes you just decide that what was a wonderful place is now just another assault on your sanity and you have to get out of there. I moved back to South Dakota and the story continues.

Chapter 3

South Dakota is a wonderful place, full of people who are damned independent and who have a no-nonsense way of handling things. This is true for the agricultural as well as the commercial sectors. It shocked me that this was, or is, also true for the medical facilities I worked in. Well, not so much the facility, but the people who made up the staff of the facility.

My first day on the job at a small hospital in the Black Hills in the western part of the state was quite uneventful. I met the people I would be working with and learned the layout of the department. The people were nice, although a couple seemed to be a little strange. I met Leila and Pat. The other names escape me because these are the two people that caught my attention the most. Leila was a woman about five or six years older than me, and was very pleasant to talk to and be around. Pat was a CRNA (certified registered nurse anesthetist) and he gave new meaning to the word, 'squirrelly'. He was a slender, nervous man who never shut up. I really believe that when he dies the family will mount a speaker on his coffin so he can chatter for all eternity.

Leila showed me around the hospital and took me down to the cafeteria for lunch. After we filled our trays with food we headed for a table to eat. She looked me dead in the eyes and said, "Run. Run away from here as fast as you can. This place is totally insane." She then stabbed a potato and ate it.

Taken a little bit by surprise I stuttered, "Leila I have worked in insanity before as a combat medic. It can't be that bad here, can it?"

She just shrugged and ate her lunch. I followed suit and after we finished we headed back up to the operating room. The first few days were uneventful, but as we know that is normally the lull before the storm. I was feeling comfortable having done a few cases with the surgeons and everything was going well. I was getting ready to do an orthopedic procedure when Leila walked up and said, "He is an asshole don't let him buffalo you." She turned and walked away and I was left wondering how this surgeon's personality would manifest itself. It didn't take long to find out.

I had everything set up for the procedure when Doctor Skip walked in, looked around the room, and grunted. He turned his attention to me and demanded, "Who the hell are you, and what are you doing in my room? I want Dan."

Looking him in the eye I replied, "I am Micheal, and Dan isn't here." I turned to my back table and ignored him. Pat had finished putting the patient to sleep and we prepped the patient's leg and started the draping procedure. Skip would hold out his hand and snap what he wanted. I would hand it to him and he would use it. He held out his hand and snapped, "Roll." I handed him a six-inch bias roll. He looked in his hand glared at me, and proceeded to throw the bias on the floor and scream, "You ignorant fool! You don't know what a roll is?" He pointed at a roll of towels which is called a 'bump' in every surgery room but his.

I looked at the bump and then looked on the floor at the roll of bias. He was turning red and getting ready for another outburst when I casually stated, "You wanted a bump, not a roll. If you don't know the names of things just ask and I will tell you. And another thing, you are acting pretty damned immature throwing stuff on the floor; you need a good spanking if you ask me."

There was absolute silence in the room. Pat was hiding behind the anesthesia machine, the nurse, Lucy, was sitting rigidly still in her chair, and I was thinking that I could get a job at the hospital in Sturgis. Skip looked at me, looked at the bias on the floor, and started to laugh. Then he thumped me in the chest and said, "I like you." The rest of my time there I could do no wrong with Skip. We talked hunting, fishing, and shooting during our cases. I even had a standing invitation to come to his ranch anytime to hunt or fish.

It was during one of our discussions in a case that I learned Pat was called Prairie Dog, because he would pop up every couple of minutes and look over the drape then pop back down. This would go on during the entire case and could be very annoying after a while. One day Skip asked me, "Do you like prairie dog hunting?"

I replied, "Yeah, it's challenging." Skip took a clean lap sponge and soaked it in saline. He placed it on the mayo stand and we went back to work. Just like clockwork, up popped Pat, but before he could drop down again, Skip grabbed the sponge and threw it, catching Pat in the forehead. He then turned to me and said, "I like prairie dog hunting too, especially in the OR." I couldn't help it, I cracked up laughing until it hurt.

Leila was amazed that Skip and I were getting along and that he was friendly and polite to me. I explained about our first meeting and she nodded and walked away. I was not sure what had transpired and decided that it was something that would be clear at some point.

Leila is a wonderful human being and an excellent nurse. A kinder, more loving person would be difficult to find. That is the one side of Leila, but like most of us, Leila has a dark side too. I had the privilege to be in the operating room when this side emerged. I will admit, spending time with her family on picnics and fishing trips allowed me to get to know her and find out something about her past. Juan, her husband, is Chilean by birth but now is a proud American citizen. He and I would be fly fishing along one of the rivers in the area and he would tell me stories of how he met 'Lei' as he called her. Here her background, as I received it, and it should give you some understanding of why things happened as they did in two very specific instances, involving two very difficult surgeons:

Leila was raised on a ranch about twenty miles from the one I was raised on. She learned to ride, shoot, butcher, and use a knife proficiently, as she was one of five daughters on the ranch. There were no sons, so the girls learned to do all that needed to be done to help out on the ranch. When Leila graduated high school, she received a scholarship to a local nursing school and decided that would be a great career. She graduated top of her class and immediately took a position in Chile as a missionary nurse at a remote hospital.

There were sporadic revolutions going on at some place or the other in the country at that time, and one day, according to Juan, a local revolutionary leader and a dozen of his men came into the area and immediately went to the hospital, demanding that all the patients leave so his men could rest and relax as they recovered from minor wounds suffered in the life of a revolutionary. Leila was in charge of the hospital and went to talk with the leader. Juan said Leila flatly told the leader that her patients were not going to be put out, but that she and her nurses would take care of his wounded, injured, and sick. The leader said, "Of course you will, now remove the other patients."

Leila said, "I will treat everyone, or no one your choice." That was the end of the discussion and nobody had to leave the hospital. A few days later Leila went to the leader and said, "Your people are bothering my nurses and this must stop."

The leader just laughed and asked Leila, "Who am I to interfere with nature taking its course?"

Leila just smiled and said, "Yes, who are you to interfere." The next night two of the leader's finest tried to convince a young nurse to let them enjoy her charms. She was crying and fighting a losing battle when first one and then the other attacker looked stunned, and fell to the ground bleeding. The young nurse ran crying into the darkness. The next day the leader was livid and called for hostages to be taken and executed if the person who attacked his men did not come forward.

Leila went to the leader and said, "No hostages will be taken. Your men are not dead and they are being taken care of in the hospital. You would be better off controlling your men since there is a good chance they could be more than wounded next time."

"Are you threatening my men?" he demanded

Leila just smiled and replied, "Why, no Commander. I am just telling of human nature and how things can spiral out of control if one is not careful."

Things were quiet for a week or so and then a young nurse was raped and murdered by a revolutionary. Witnesses identified the man to Leila and she went to the leader to get this taken care of once and for all. The leader just laughed at her and ordered her out of the office. Two days later there was the sound of a shot on the hillside and when people arrived they found the rapist/murderer dead with a bullet in his brain. The leader went ballistic and started to shout and threaten everyone. His second in command was trying to calm him down saying that the man was a pig and deserved what had happened to him, and that the leader knew it was true. However, the leader would not listen to the man and stomped off to write the orders to take hostages. Juan says Leila walked over and asked the second in command what he would do if he were the leader and the young man said, "I would leave and take the men home to their families and their crops." Later that day the leader died mysteriously and the second in command lead his men home.

Several weeks later, Leila was assigned to an orthopedic case with Skip and me. She never worked with Skip, and I really don't know how she managed that. Today was the day for her time in the mix. One needs to understand that Skip treated nurses like they were second class people. He would make them stand in the corner so they would not distract him during surgery. On this day, we were doing an arthroscopy and Skip was a real pain in the ass when he was using a scope. He would go into a rage if the nurse moved around when he was scoping. He said it made him sea-sick to have that back-ground movement. During this case Leila had to move some equipment and Skip went off on her as he pulled his gloves off and stormed over. He grabbed her by the shoulders and pushed her into the corner yelling, "You stand there until I tell you to move." He put on another pair of gloves and we finished the case. Leila, in the meantime, moved back over to her desk to do charting. Skip saw it, but just grumbled. The case was over and we prepared to leave the room. I was looking at Leila and saw something in her eyes that gave me pause.

Skip was walking towards the door and as he got close, Leila stood up and stepped in front of him. He stopped and looked at her as she grabbed him by the shoulders and slammed him against the wall. His expression was one of pure shock; being manhandled was clearly not something he was used to. He started to say something, but Leila told him to shut up. Then she talked to him in a very cold voice. "If you ever touch me again I will do things to you that will make your worst and wildest nightmares seem like happy places. Do you understand me, Skip? I will hurt you beyond imagination." She then turned from Skip and looked over at me, giving me a smile that made me believe her every word.

Strangely enough, Leila and I became the permanent team for Skip after that, with laughter and jokes and of course, prairie dog hunting.

Skip received a scare from Leila, but one other doctor was shaken to his inner core when he tried to play games with her. We were doing a bowel resection on a very obese lady and the doctor who fancied himself as the world's greatest practical joker was in rare form. The patient weighed in the excess of four hundred pounds and was not tall, so basically, she resembled a ball. As we worked to resect her bowel, we were forced to move huge amounts of fat and omenteum. In the process of removing eighteen inches of bowel, we took a very large amount of the fat around it. Our practical joker kept looking at the omenteum on the bowel and made his fateful decision. Taking the bovie, he sliced off a large piece of the fat then turned towards Leila and tossed it at her. It hit her in the chest and when she looked up in shocked surprise he told her, "Have that sent to the lab for fat analysis." With that said, he returned his attention to the patient and started to hum a happy little tune.

Leila never said a word. She put on gloves, picked the fat tissue up, and placed it in a container. She then left the room for a few minutes to change and wash up from the fat bomb thrown by the doctor. With this finished, she returned to the room and resumed her charting on the procedure. Not one word was said to the doctor about his prank.

The case went on, as all cases do, to the end. We closed the wound and made sure all the drains were in place and secure. When the dressings were applied, anesthesia woke the patient enough to be transported to a recovery room. Our doctor congratulated himself on his great skill and started to leave the room when Leila stepped in front of him and stated, "The fat analysis is back from the lab, Doctor."

The practical joker looked at her and asked, "What would the analysis be then, Leila?"

She reached up and grabbed the front of his scrub top and pulled him towards her. When he was positioned as she wanted, she drove her knee into his crotch with a force that made me have sympathy pains. The practical joker dropped to the floor in a fetal position, tears streaming from his eyes and vomit on the floor in front of him. Leila knelt down and whispered, "The lab says if you ever do any stupid games like that again, I will end your existence in the most painful way you can imagine. Do you understand what I am telling you, Doctor? I mean, do you really understand that I will not tolerate this to ever happen again?"

The practical joker just nodded his head, not even able to grunt an answer. Leila looked him in the eye and smiled that smile I had seen once before, and I knew he understood what she meant.

Nothing came of the incident. No one said anything and no one complained. Things were more pleasant in the department when the practical jokes stopped.

We had a lady working in our sterile supply department who stated routinely that she knew more about what a tech did in surgery than any tech did about what she did in sterile supply. Two of us were military trained to be techs and this training included three months, out of twelve every year, in the sterile supply department. So, after a while we became tired of hearing the brags and bravado from her. I will call her Ruth, for no better reason than it's a nice name for this annoying person. Dale, the other military trained tech, and I discussed Ruth and decided that she could use a reality check. We talked to our boss and he agreed to assign Dale and me to the sterile supply and bring her in to do a few days of simple cases. She was ecstatic about being able to teach us how it should be done. We, on the other hand, thought it would be nice to see things wrapped and assembled correctly. Dale and I had no problem organizing the sterile supply to our liking, and we showed people how we liked the sterile packs to be wrapped, how one was supposed to disassemble instruments for the sterilizing process, and how to package them in the trays.

Life was not quite so idyllic in the operating room. While Ruth knew what the equipment was and what sets it came in, she didn't quite understand sterile technique, or how to gown and glove herself and the members of the crew. With no knowledge of setup and no knowledge of what the case involved, she was lost and the doctors were quickly losing patience having to teach her everything. It was shortly after the third case that Ruth came back to the sterile supply in tears. Despite our great urge to gloat, we didn't.

When we asked her what the problem was, between sobs she related how she had always wanted to be a scrub tech. We told her there were programs available that could teach her. That's when we found out she had applied to a couple but didn't have a high school diploma, so they would not accept her. She could get into college without one but not a tech program.

We hatched a plan and conned our boss into letting us train Ruth on her days off in surgery so she could learn how to be a tech. Over the next year everyone got involved and helped. The doctors would explain what they were doing and why and what she should expect. The nurses would help with sterile technique and we, the techs, would teach her what she wanted to learn so badly. Long story short, over the course of a year with everyone helping, Ruth was able to fill a vacancy that occurred, it was mine I was going to help build and open a surgery center in the area and they offered me too much money for my knowledge, so I left.

The surgery center was the weirdest and most bizarre place I have ever worked..

When I started at the surgery center it was not completed and I had to take up hammer and nail to assist in the process to have our grand opening. We were designed with six operating rooms and twelve recovery room beds. Somehow in the licensing for the facility we received permission to have overnight stays for our patients, so there were six overnight rooms also. The surgery center would do outpatient surgeries from podiatry to micro-discectomies.

Our director of nursing was not the most tightly wound person in the world. When I say I helped to build this surgery center, I mean physically and wrote policy and procedures. Instrument ordering fell on my shoulders and so the phone calls started. The owners of the center gave me the responsibility to procure all the equipment and instrumentation needed for the center to start. They said, "You have more years of experience than any other person here. You know the surgeries we plan to do, so you can order from whoever you want, just get the best deals." So the next thing to do was to see what each instrument provider had to offer me and my three hundred and seventy-five thousand dollar budget. I told each company the same thing - I have the money and the authority, you have to offer the best deal or I will shop elsewhere. This budget didn't include the money for two microscopes and x-ray equipment.

Each company would send me a list with the proposed instrumentation and the cost. No one seemed to understand that I am cheap and when I say offer me a deal, I mean a deal! Finally, I requested that the top three companies send reps to me that week.

When the reps arrived I sat them down and told them exactly what I wanted, what I was willing to pay, and what I expected from them in return. After several hours, we came to terms and for every three sets I would purchase they would throw in a fourth one for free. In the process, I got the neuro instruments, the orthopedic instruments, and the general instruments for the center. Podiatry, dental, and ENT instruments were negotiated with the specialty companies, and in the end, I returned seventy-four thousand dollars to the center.

In the beginning the other two techs, one nurse, and I would sit down and look at the surgery schedule for the following day. We would then decide how to put together the sets needed for the next day. As each case was discussed we put together the set and made up a temp card for the procedure. Since it was my responsibility to do the computer work for cards, sets, and cases, I would stay over, typing it all into the system. After a while we let the people who do the sterilization actually do their job and we stopped washing and assembling the instruments as our system became more efficient and the instruments became standardized.

Some items we didn't buy, mainly because we would only use them one or two times a year. During those times the rep for the company would send us the instruments we needed for the procedure. In theory that works wonderfully, however in practice, it does not. Part of my responsibility was to get in touch with the rep when we needed instruments for a case the next week. However, as I mentioned earlier, my director of nurses was not too tightly wound. She told me that she would take care of ordering sets because it was not my place to do managerial duties. I asked if she needed me to help with what we had to have and was told, "You are a tech, I am the DON, you really don't think I need your advice, do you?" I was tempted to say 'Yes, I think you do', but I held my tongue.

Later that day she told me that my instruments would be here the first of the week and I really needed to stop worrying. I thought nothing more about it and went about my duties. The case was scheduled for the following Friday and so we had time to get in all the extras that were needed.

On Monday, the instruments didn't show up, nor did they arrive the next day, or the next, or the one after that. I questioned the DON about the instruments and she told me she was taking care of it and that I should just do my job. So, on Friday at eight in the morning, the instruments arrived; our case was scheduled for ten that morning. A very proud and arrogant DON wheeled the instruments into the setup room and, smirking, said, "I told you I was handling it." She then turned on her heel and strutted out of the room. The circulating nurse and I opened the boxes so we could inventory and check the sets before sterilizing them. Instead of the two pans of instruments for the procedure there was only one, and after closer inspection we discovered that half the instruments we needed were missing. Further inspection showed that the joint shaver and attachments were for an ankle, not a knee, and was not interchangeable.

I took the sets to the DON and showed her what was missing and why we were screwed if I couldn't find the correct sets. She immediately started to scream at me for my negativity and demanded an explanation for why I could not do the case with the instruments in the set. I showed her how one part of an instrument was needed to be used in conjunction with another, but since I was missing those ancillary pieces we just couldn't do the case. In a panic, she fled the room, calling the surgeon's name.

As she was telling the doctor that the case couldn't be done, I was getting my address book from my locker and calling a friend in the business. I told him what happened and asked if he could help us out. He said he would since I had gotten him into the surgery center with some orthopedic implants his company sold. Twenty minutes before the case was to start my friend Brad came in with complete sterilized instrument sets and the proper shaver and tips, all sterile, and I threw them on a cart, called the room tech and said, "Set it up."

I was talking to Brad when the doctor came up and started to chastise me about not ordering the proper instruments, adding that he wondered if they were paying me too much since I didn't seem to have the ability to get the job done properly. Brad turned to the doctor and proceeded to explain that I got everything that was needed for the case and how the doctor's tech was opening it as we spoke. The doctor looked at me and demanded to know why I didn't get it right the first time. I asked the doctor if he would do me a favor and if it showed that I was incompetent I would resign from the facility.

He agreed so I called the rep the DON arranged everything with and told the doctor to ask him why Hopkins blew the order so badly. He asked and the rep said, "I never talked to Hopkins. I talked to the DON and she said she was handling all the special ordering now."

The doctor just looked at me then turned and walked away. I don't know what was said in the DON's office, but shortly after he talked to her I was told that I would now do all the ordering of extra instruments for procedures.

As I stated earlier we were in the process of building and opening the surgery center and the DON oversaw many policies and procedures. One of her pet projects was our disaster and emergency alert system. Most people are familiar with Code Blue, Code Red, Code Brown, etc. She did not want that system at the surgery center, fearing that patients and family would freak out if they were to hear such calls over the intercom system. She decided to model our emergency call system after characters in the Wizard of Oz. Code Blue was now Code Tinman, Code Red was now Code Strawman, and a lost child was

Code Dorothy. She designed her perfect system, had wonderful plastic laminated cards and placards made up, and even hired a local artist to paint the characters on the wall of the office with the code under them. It all would have been very nice if one ran a daycare. When she turned her project into the board of directors for final approval and showed the cards, placards, and artwork to the same board, it was rejected and called stupid. The board was made up of doctors who invested in the surgery center and wanted to make money not waste it on, as they put it, "Stupid assed projects to reinvent a perfectly good wheel."

I moved on to another local hospital after the DON started to find strange fault with me. I was written up because I used words that seemed "too fancy" and this made the nurses feel I was talking down to them. I said, "Okay, no problem, I can solve that issue without delay."

One month later I was written up because I was not interacting with my co-workers and only responded to them with 'Yes', 'No', or some pleasantry. I would say 'Good Morning', 'Good

Afternoon', and 'Good Night'. If I asked a nurse for something I would say what I needed and then thank them for getting it. I entered no conversations or initiated any. When I received this write up I said, "You can't have it both ways, either I talk or I don't and I will not apologize for the level of language I use, because that is what I learned growing up." She was offended and threatened me with suspension. I smiled and handed her my written resignation, dated that day, and walked out the door.

Prior to my trip to her office I knew what was coming down so I went to the computers and removed all the programs I had written and put into the system. The inventory, the worksheets for cases, and the entire program I had written to do negative entry billing. These were mine. I did them at home, on my time, and on my equipment, using my programs, that I owned. I never said a word about I and it was a week or so later that I received a phone call from one of the secretaries who wanted to know why she couldn't enter the billing program. I asked her what billing program she was talking about and hung up.

Chapter 4

The next hospital I went to work at was also part of a huge healthcare network, but it seemed to be the poor red-headed stepchild. If you needed something, you put in several requisitions and then made phone calls begging the materials management director for the supplies. She would never give you anything you wanted until the second begging phone call. At some point, she irritated someone enough that there was a phone call to the police about drugs in her car. She was fired because the healthcare system didn't want any trouble or bad press, and would fire their own grandmother to save face. The new materials person was more amenable to getting us what we needed

We had a small operating suite in this hospital, as in, we had one OR and one procedure room. When I started there, they had one nurse/scrub and she was a stickler for PAR levels. She was not much of a stickler for what went on during surgery, however. I was informed that this nurse could do three of the same procedures in a row and would need to be retrained for the start of the next one.

Another interesting factor was turn over time for the rooms was a minimum of one hour. Doctors would wander off to do clinic or have lunch between cases. When I started with my old nurse from the surgery center as my RN, we did our own turnovers in ten minutes and would call the surgeon to come back, because we were ready to go. The slow nurse argued that the doctors wanted the delay so they could take care of business. We asked the docs if that was true and they just laughed and said, "What, are you brain damaged? We begged for faster turnover times for years and were stonewalled."

We did some heavy cases at this little hospital with one operating room and one procedure room. We did bowel resections and different vascular cases, including Triple A's. We had three surgeons that were extremely talented and they would do miracles when it came to surgery. Unfortunately, the other scrub tech was not up to the talent of our surgeons. I remember one cold, snowy night my phone rang at two in the morning and when I answered one of the doctors said, "I am doing a Triple A in thirty minutes, so hurry down."

I stated, "Um, Uncle Larry, I am not on call, Lynn is."

He responded, "I know, but I want the patient to live, so please get your lazy ass out of bed and get down here."

So out into the cold and snow I went, to drive the thirteen miles to the hospital. Upon arrival, I saw my friend Ron was there and we threw a room together for a Triple A. Lynn was there also, not helping, just watching. Ron and I had the room open in five minutes and I scrubbed in and set up. I have a quick setup for dead serious emergency cases, it involves throwing the entire instrument stringer on the mayo stand and counting it, then pulling back what I won't need. This took another five minutes and Lynn was just standing with her hands in her pockets, yawning. I asked if she wanted to learn anything. She turned on her heel and went home. I told Ron she had to go and he agreed.

During the winter, we worked to rid ourselves of Lynn and after finding there was a place open for her in materials, we convinced her she would be doing so much more good for the system and she could monitor Par levels hospital wide. She jumped at the chance.

In early spring, we found a fart machine. It was left in a storage room in surgery and we figured that it would be a perfect addition to our program of passive annoyance around the hospital. One of our doctors was a very prim, and therefore, annoying man. We slipped the fart machine into his lab coat pocket along with all the other "important" stuff he carried in his coat. He had requested Ron and I accompany him on his rounds of the surgical patients he had in house. So, we agreed and placed the machine. I had the remote for it in my lab coat pocket as we set out.

The very first person we ran into on the tour was the secretary for the hospital administrator. She stopped the doctor to tell him of an upcoming meeting and wanted his input. As he was opening his mouth to answer, I pressed the button and released a short blat of sound from the area of the doctor. The secretary looked shocked and backed up a step. Mr. Prim Doctor didn't seem to notice the sound and stepped closer to tell her his thoughts, when I set off a chain of farts ending with one that sort of faded away. The secretary turned on her heel and fled. Doctor Prim turned to us and said, "She really should cut down on her roughage, it's making her very flatulent." We bit our tongues and nodded in agreement.

Continuing down the hall we passed our X-ray tech, and as the doctor acknowledged her greeting I fired off the device again.

She looked at him and said, "Well, I am waiting."

The doctor asked, "For what are you waiting?"

She responded, "For your apology over breaking wind in my presence."

Our doctor looked stunned and stuttered, "That wasn't me young lady, you are mistaken." He kept shaking his head as we continued down the hall towards his patient's room. Ron and I kept silent and tried our best to not laugh out loud over his discomfort. Arriving at the room where his patient was recuperating from surgery, we noticed a very rotund man with red cheeks and a huge smile. The doctor greeted his patient and asked how he was doing.

"Doing great Doc; absolutely fantastic," was the man's response. "As a matter of fact, I think I can go home today."

"Why would you say that, Arthur? It's only two days post-op and you know we have to get your bowels functioning again. You have to pass some gas…" As the doctor said this the patient let out a long and impressive fart.

"Well Doc how was that?" Before he could answer I held the button down on the fart machine and it sounded like a drum roll. The doctor looked shocked. Finally realization registered on his face, and he looked at me and growled, "If you have anything at all to do with this I expect you to end it now. Do I make myself clear?"

Ron started to laugh and reached into the lab coat, pulling out the fart machine. The patient laughed. "Is that what I think it is? I just pushed the button in response. The doctor turned beet red and said, "Out now, get out!"

We took off running laughing the whole way. As we rounded the corner we heard Doctor Prim laughing with his patient. Nothing more was said over the incident.

The fart machine did not disappear, we used it one more time. One bright and sunny day we decided that our anesthesia provider, Bubba, was taking himself and his position too seriously, so we put the machine to use. Before our big case of the day started we, (read that as I) taped the fart machine to the underside of his anesthesia throne. He thought he was the king of the operating room so we had already labeled the chair 'the Throne of Bubba'. He liked that and had a brass plaque made up and attached to his chair.

Everything was ready for the case and the remote for the machine was attached to the waist of my scrubs, within easy reach. The case started and only three people knew what was about to happen: the circulator, my boss Ron, who was the second scrub, and myself. The surgeons had no knowledge of what was to happen, and for sure, neither did Bubba. As per his habit, Bubba was giving his opinion on every news item, rumor, gossip, or hearsay item that caught his attention. We all knew his opinions because we all suffered through them daily. Today if the gods were kind to us we would have our revenge. Bubba started in on the local hospital gossip about one of the administrators allegedly having an affair with a nurse. True to Bubba, he paraphrased his next statement with the words, "You wanna know what I think? I think that they should…" it was at this moment the fart machine fired off a long burst of sound. Bubba looked totally shocked and yelled, "Hey that wasn't me! The gas machine just hiccoughed."

To which one of the surgeons replied, "Yeah that was a gas machine I heard. What did you have for lunch, Bubba?"

Bubba emphatically replied, "I said that wasn't me!" I looked at Ron, he was turning red and the circulator was wiping tears from her eyes. Bubba continued to look thoroughly offended that someone could accuse him of such a plebian act as farting.

Things calmed down and Bubba started in on another subject that needed his noble input. It seemed that local politicians had been caught doing what politicians do - interfering with people's lives and businesses. The locals wanted to annex part of a local rancher's land into the city for a new public works project site. The rancher was upset. What Bubba and the others didn't know was the identity of the rancher, because the story had not completely unfolded yet. I knew who the rancher was because I hunted with him to control varmints that preyed on young calves. He was also one of the surgeons on staff at the hospital. He swore me to secrecy over the ongoing situation. So, I was interested to hear what Bubba had to say, but still more interested in embarrassing him. Bubba puffed up and announced that, "It is a citizen's duty to assist the government in times of need and to help those who have less than others."

One of the surgeons asked, "So you believe the government can just come in and take a citizen's property?"

Bubba nodded his head and stated, "When it is in the best interest of the people, I think that the government is mandated to…" Another click of the button and his explanation was drowned out by the sweet sound of gas expulsion. Bubba jumped out of his chair and started to rant, "Someone better confess to passing gas when I am talking!" We all looked shocked, well, the doctors looked genuinely shocked and Ron, the circulator, and I looked as shocked as we could while trying not to laugh out loud.

One of the surgeons asked Bubba, "Did you go to the Uncle Larry School of Social Graces?" Uncle Larry being notorious for his farts during surgery. Bubba started to protest, but one of the doctors asked him if the patient was doing okay and this shut him down. Bubba sat back down, but every time he would move his chair a fart followed. We would look at him and ask if he could cut back on the air assault. He swore it wasn't him, it had to be the anesthesia machine needing some sort of adjustment; he then busied himself with gauges, knobs, and switches for the next ten minutes. As he made each adjustment he would turn to his patient's monitor, and with each turn the button was pushed, and he turned redder and redder.

The attending surgeon looked over the barrier between the operative field and Bubba's area and said, "Bubba you are aware that the term we use for your position is not literal, it is about your anesthetic gases; not the gas from your colon?" We all started to laugh and Bubba emphatically denied that he had any connection to the farting sounds and blamed his machine once again. To which, the assistant surgeon said, "A good craftsman does not blame his tools."

Bubba went ballistic and the fart machine rumbled and roared in time to his anger and frustration. I heard an "Oh damn" and turned to see the circulator had wet herself from laughing so hard at Bubba's discomfort. Ron was sitting on the floor laughing as tears rolled down his cheeks. I maintained my dignity and kept my finger on the fart machine remote.

The case eventually ended with Bubba calling medical equipment repair to get into the OR ASAP and fix his farting anesthesia machine. The surgeons offered to write Bubba a prescription for anti-gas medications, and Bubba was not talking to anyone any more. As the case closed and Bubba started to extubate the patient, I ended his pain with one long blast of the machine. After the case, when the patient and anesthesia were on their way to the recovery room, I went over to Bubba's throne and removed the fart machine. As I turned to leave I found that the attending surgeon was standing in the door way with a huge grin on his face. "I thought the farts sounded too consistent," he said, "Give me that thing so I can use it in the office tomorrow and I won't tell Bubba."

I handed it to him with a laugh and asked, "Did you see the circulator pee herself laughing?"

To which he replied, "I was worried that Ron was going to fall over and hit his head as he sat on the floor." I never saw the fart machine again but I heard that it was making the rounds.

Being a scrub tech is not all glamour and good times, you have to stay until the cases are done, you must stand for long hours, and you must come to work in all kinds of weather and all hours of the day or night. I was called in one night at midnight by Uncle Larry, to do an emergency foreign body removal from a man's esophagus. My second youngest son was awake and asked how long the case would take. I said, "With Uncle Larry, no more than half an hour. Why?"

He told me he was bored and wanted something to do because sleep was not in the mix yet. So, if I didn't mind he would drive me to work and wait. We had just finished a brake job and some minor transmission work on his car, so I agreed, thinking we might as well give it a test drive.

Walking outside our house I noticed it was snowing and we already had eight or ten inches on the ground with no let up in sight for the near future. We took off and were soon on the shortest route from our house to the hospital. The snow was coming down hard, but the road itself was very slushy with melted snow that lacked the ambition to become ice. We were about half-way there when for some reason the car broke traction and began a slow three hundred and sixty degree turn, but hitting something a little harder in the roadway caused the car to slide backwards, towards a twenty-five foot drop-off into the woods. My son looked scared. I told him in a calm voice, "Don't touch the brakes and don't turn your wheel."

"When I tell you to I want you to slam the throttle to the floor and gently turn your wheels to the left." He just looked at me blankly, and I said, "Trust me."

I was looking out the back window and said, "Do it now!" He slammed his foot to the floor and turned the steering wheel. The car surged forward and back onto the road. He stopped the car and we walked back to see we had about two inches before the rear tires would have gone off the edge of the road and into the woods below.

My son was smiling like there was nothing wrong in the world. "Dad, you knew that the car would go into four-wheel drive if I spun the rear wheels, didn't you?" I smiled and said, "Yup." He then reached into my pocket pulled out my cigarettes, and lite one up. I gave him a questioning look and he just grinned and said, "I know I don't smoke and I don't allow it in the car, but come on, this is the second time you have saved our bacon with calmness and no yelling." So, we had a smoke on the way to work.

I walked in and Uncle Larry asked, "What the hell are you doing here on a night like this?" I told him the charge nurse had called me in. "Well then, punch in and go home. I'll punch you out when I am done," he said.

I laughed and told him it was okay, I would stay and help. We started to anesthetize the patients throat when he started to gag, and he gagged so hard that he vomited up the obstruction - a large unchewed piece of pork chop. He was drunk, and drunks have a problem chewing completely when they are eating. Uncle Larry did a quick look with the scope and we were done. I cleaned the scope, left it in the soak for the remainder of the night and went home with my son. We drove back more cautiously than our initial trip.

We had a general practitioner who thought that he was the be all end all of C-section surgeries. Every time one of his patients needed to have a C-section, he would be right there taking the place of someone who was competent and skilled. However, being that the patients were his, he became the assistant surgeon. We all did our best to keep him from hurting himself or killing someone. He had this fetish that whenever you were to do a C-section the tech needed to have hot lap sponges for the case. We never gave them to him and would ignore his constant demands for them. He would take a regular lap sponge, and every time the surgeon would stop the bleeding the assistant would rub the site vigorously with the sponge and start the bleeding again. We would allow him to do this three times and then we would remove his sponge and refuse to return it. The case would continue to the end, he would get paid for doing nothing, and we were happy to keep him from killing patients.

One case this general practitioner would do without a watch dog doctor was a D&C.

It was an early afternoon and the doctor called us to come in for a D&C on a young lady who had delivered several hours before, but was still bleeding. He believed that she had some retained placenta. We started the case and he was scraping and suctioning to get all the remaining placenta out and she continued to bleed. The doctor was now starting to talk about an emergency hysterectomy and I was starting to think he had over-looked something.

Taking a wild shot in the dark I asked the doctor, "Sir, do you think a second dose of Vasopressin would help?" I really believed that he didn't give the initial dose, but felt it was more diplomatic to ask in the way I did. He looked at me strangely and then told the anesthesia provider, who happened to be Bubba, to give a second dose of Vasopressin to the patient.

Bubba, not as diplomatic as me, said, "You never ordered the first dose, so this will be an initial dose." The drug was given and within a couple minutes the bleeding stopped and we were done.

The doctor turned to me and said, "Don't ever presume to tell me or to suggest to me a treatment for one of my patients. If you do it again, I will have you fired." I smiled and told him it would not be a problem because the next time I would just let nature take its course and then advise, anonymously to sue his slimy ass for malpractice." Strangely enough we never exchanged Christmas cards.

A year after I left the hospital a patient of his died through his ministrations of poor medical practice. It was shortly after that when I was offered a job in Michigan. I took it and entered the world that sanity forgot.

Michigan is a lovely state. The people are, for the most part, friendly and have a good sense of humor. The weather is a mixture of pleasant to frigid to scorching to dripping humidity inter-spaced with an occasional snow fall. The people of Michigan are survivors - they don't commit suicide because of the lack of sunlight, they don't generally rise in mass and riot; however, when they do they do it surprisingly well… burning their inner cities to ashes. Generally, it's just a day to day working class state.

I moved to an area with a state university full of young minds seeking knowledge, beer, pot, and parties; they were having fun and pretending to get an education. I need to describe the hospital as a structure to give you an idea of what lay ahead. When the facility was built they assumed that cars were not really going to be a big thing (remember this was in the auto building capital of the United States). So, for a facility of two hundred thirty-six beds they had parking for roughly that many cars. The hospital bought all the houses on one side of the facility, promising to not tear them down but to use them for offices and housing for temporary help. Someone in the administration figured that with the eleven homes they bought, the facility could make some serious money utilizing the property. One day the bulldozers came in and seven of the houses disappeared under the tracks to become a big vacant lot that was used to store construction equipment for a local contractor. The remaining neighbors complained and threatened to sue for violation of contract. The hospital backed down, paved over the entire area, and put up signs, fences and card key gates. But they never used the area for anything at all.

This is the place I came to call home for eight long crazy years. My wife and I had a great apartment in a relatively nice area. We overlooked the pool and the moonlight on the skinny dippers after the pool closed didn't do much to make them look any better. The management was benign and maintenance was prompt and efficient if they liked you. We always had beer in the fridge for the maintenance people and they would stop in just to see if we needed something fixed. Sometimes the inspection was two beers long.

My first day at the hospital the manager introduced me to the other staff and physicians and anyone who happened to be wandering through the area. The staff was pretty much what you would expect at a community hospital. There were three bullies, all female, another male who thought he was a war hero, and an assortment of doctors that covered a broad spectrum of talents, skills, and abilities.

I met one CRNA who became a longtime friend and is now my best friend in the world. I met others who were talented and caring and then I met the assistant anesthesiologist. When I say assistant, I mean he was the junior partner in a two-man office and was a real nut case. He was, for the most part, harmless and pleasant. However, he had a wandering eye, wandering hands, and a tendency to lie to the staff to get a patient into the room. He also had an Italian wife from New York who, it was rumored, was in 'the family' or, the mob. Our doctor lived in cringing fear of upsetting his wife. Who knows, he may have ended up sleeping with the fishes if he did. Anyway, the doc, who I will call Joe, was always trying to impress the CRNA staff with his prowess as an anesthetist. The CRNAs would listen, nod their heads politely, and continue to do what they were doing. But before I go too far let me say that I have seen no one better when it came to anesthesia for a new born or very young infant. Unfortunately, his skills, combined with his annoying personality, combined with his ego, didn't help with everyday cases. We had a locums CRNA come in to the facility to fill an opening when one of the other full time CRNAs left for greener pastures, with less Joe to distract them. I was in the operating room when he was brought in by Joe and introduced to the staff. I was looking at this man and he was staring at me. Joe asked, if there a problem between us that he wasn't aware of?

Ignoring him, I asked; the new locums, "Were you at Dakota Wesleyan University in 68?"

"Yeah just out of Vietnam and the marines going to nursing school."

I started to laugh and asked him, "Are you that crazy Indian from Kadoka?"

He laughed "You were that longhaired, drug crazed, hippy cowboy from the west river!"

I said, "Yup how you been, Lee?"

He just smiled and told me we would talk after the case. By this time Joe was totally confused and asked me, "Are you a drug addict? And do you need to be tested to continue your employment at the hospital?" I just laughed and told him to go screw himself and that I would drug test when he did.

The hospital I worked at was different in so many ways. It was almost inbred in the administration, with current or former lovers, spouses, and significant others all occupying the top positions. Intrigue and slapstick comedy in the making. The administrator was a former lab employee who was fired for embezzlement. He went to school, received his degree in Hospital Administration, and for some strange reason was hired as the CEO of the hospital.

We had a psych ward at the hospital that was run by a psychiatrist from Georgia. The hospital would fly him in weekly, first class for him and his dog. They would put him up in the Holiday Inn and pay him five hundred thousand dollars a year to work three days a week. He would get eight weeks of paid vacation a year and unlimited personal days off with pay. I guess there were no psychiatrists living in Michigan that would work at the hospital. The average census for the psych ward was three patients. But the ward had twenty-seven nurses working in it so it must have been dangerous. If they had any problems when the director was back in Georgia the staff was told to contact the county mental health department for medication or consoling needs. The county eventually jerked the hospital's credentials to be a mental health facility and no one really noticed except the twenty-seven nurses who had to find work in the hospital or elsewhere.

I worked with a former corpsman who always wanted to compare his time in Panama with my time as a combat medic. We had a nurse who was so simple that she would fall for anything, a lesbian who had a golden personality, and the usual psychotics that you get who have worked nowhere else and had the seniority to make your life miserable. I had three techs who hated their husbands beyond measure and a lovely nurse who had an abusive husband but she didn't know she was being abused. The lesbian nurse loved this lovely nurse and would buy her teddies and skimpy underwear and invite her over for sleep overs with her and her wife. I don't know if she ever went but the gifts continued and she seemed happy.

Doctors were another matter in this hospital. I was blessed with two doctors from India who hated each other, since one was Hindu and the other Catholic. We had three gyn surgeons who were pleasant to work with and had a sense of humor. We had two orthopedic surgeons - one who was pleasant and slow and one we nick named The Prince of Darkness. We had several general surgeons who did well and one bariatric surgeon who was a hand full of uncouth.

When I walked into the surgical unit for the first time and into the break room, all conversation stopped. I was being visually dissected by everyone in the room.

One older woman stood up, walked over to me and said, "You're new here so I will tell you the way it is. I am Mrs. Sommers to you, until such time I decide to change it." She then turned around and as she was walking away, she added, "You will get call here if we don't want it, and we always want the call." She then proceeded to sit down and glare at me as though she was expecting an argument. Little did she know I hate call, I have always hated call and really would not miss it if I never pulled it again. But I knew that despite her statement I would be getting more call than I really wanted.

The next person to speak to me was the very large male tech. He laughed and said, "So finally I get to be higher in seniority than someone. Maybe the women will leave me alone and pick on you instead."

I smiled and replied, "Maybe, but I don't get picked on very well." I then asked him to show me around, because it seemed no one else was interested in anything but a very large box of doughnuts on the counter. We left and I received the fifty cent tour with anecdotes about how abused he was and how the doctors just didn't understand the real world; typical operating room complaints.

My first day was pretty much spent learning where things were and why they were there. I pulled cases for the next day and watched as Joe, (the other male scrub tech) would pull the case card and then pull the cases without using the card. I asked him why and he explained that the females had a power trip going and would not put down all the pertinent information on the case cards. They, as the old saying goes, knew that knowledge was power and if you didn't share it you were king, or in this case, queen, of the dung heap.

I said, "That's wonderful but why are you not using the cards?"

He laughed. "I memorized all the cards the first month I was here and just keep current to changes." It made sense to me because that is how I pulled cases too.

When the day was done I changed my clothes and went home.

My wife asked, "So how is it at the new hospital?"

I chuckled. "The women have dirty mouths and swear continually." We had a good laugh and then prepared a first day at the new job dinner. Basically, it was chili dogs and potato tots.

The job was pretty much boring, which in surgery, is fine. We do not like excitement in surgery. I learned the routine, pulled call, and settled in. After a few weeks Mrs. Sommers decided I could call her Karen, but I continued to call her Mrs. Sommers. When she questioned it I said, "I admire your skill and professionalism so much I think Mrs. Sommers is a perfect way to express my admiration." She was all bubbly and happy about the "compliment" I gave her.

Joe walked over and laughingly told me, "Damn boy, you could sell ice to an Eskimo with that line of bull crap."

I looked shocked and offended and purred, "Whatever could you be talking about Joe?" He slapped me on the back and knocked me halfway across the room, chuckling as he helped me set up my next case.

My first weird surgery was with our bariatric surgeon. He, as I stated earlier was a boatload of uncouth. His two favorite past times were belching the alphabet during a case and releasing huge foul-smelling farts. We were in a long case and he was talking about the great bean burritos his wife made for him the previous evening. His PA (Physician's Assistant) asked if this meant we were going to be treated to a barrage of his gaseous out puttings. He nodded and said, "Yup, starting right now." With that statement, he raised his right leg and released a huge foul-smelling fart. My nurse immediately opened a bottle of Nil Odor, it is an odor eliminating product and works well, but its limitations were being tested by the bariatric surgeon.

Our very naïve and innocent nurse walked behind the doctor, and after looking at his gown and the back side of his scrub pant legs asked, "Um are you going commando, Doctor?"

The surgeon turned. "I always go commando you want to see?" After a minute of thought the surgeon asked, "Why would you ask me something like that anyway?"

The nurse replied, "You have a huge brown stain on the back of your legs and there are little commandos on the floor." The surgeon looked down at the floor and ran from the room leaving the PA and me to close the wound. The supervisor called in and said that the rest of the surgeon's cases were canceled, and that he was going home. We had a great laugh and every time we did a procedure with him after that day the standard question was, “So Doctor, do farts have lumps?” He found no humor in our questions which was fine; we were easily amused.

It’s not hard to remember one strange surgeon or his quirks. However, this hospital was like a breeding ground for the bizarre and strange. We had two doctors from India who made the world an interesting place. I remember one of the doctors, I will call him Zack, was a short feisty little man who was always calling the women streetwalkers and not nice people. We were doing a case one afternoon, and it had been a long day of listening to him complain about everything and everyone. I remember this incident well because it really made the primary basis of our relationship almost into an adversarial one.

I handed him the syringe with local in it because our patient was showing signs of discomfort. You learn to recognize the signs of discomfort, such as, trying to climb off the table, screaming, and screams for pain medication. Our patient was exhibiting all these signs of discomfort and no matter how many times Zack told him to lay still, quit moving, and be quiet, the patient didn't cooperate. So, we injected him with Lidocaine with Epinephrine and the patient was just having none of it. He decided he was in pain and nothing short of total anesthesia would help.

Zack looked at me with a disgusted look on his face and snarled, "Why did you not give me the local I wanted?"

I looked at him and said, "I did; it's in the syringe in your right hand and you injected it."

The changing point of our relationship came with the next words he snapped at me, "You are a liar! You didn't give me what I wanted, you are just a Caucasian liar!"

I looked him in the eye and replied, "Listen you little shit! I don't lie and if I did it would not be to the likes of you, so apologize or find another tech." He refused and called me a liar again. I told the nurse to call the supervisor to come into the room. My supervisor came in and asked what the problem was.

Before I could even answer, Zack screamed, "This lying tech has given me something that is not what I asked for. He lied and is causing my patient pain and wasting my time."

My boss looked at me and asked, "What did he ask for and what did you give him?"

My reply was short and to the point, "Lido with Epi and that is what is in the syringe, in the cup, and labeled on the vial on the nurse's desk." I further explained, "I didn't pour it, Martha did, and we confirmed what it was by the label. We checked expiration dates, and verified it was unopened until she opened it."

My boss went over picked up the bottle examined it, and turned to the doctor. "Zack, you owe Micheal an apology. This bottle verifies what he stated and it was opened in accordance to protocols. So, apologize."

Zack just snarled, "He is a liar! I don't want him in my cases until he admits to his deception."

I looked at my boss and in a calm voice stated, "Darla I want to file a complaint against the doctor for insulting language and making for a hostile work environment."

She smiled and said, "I will get someone to come in and take over the case, and will pour him a new local that he can check himself and then we will go do the paperwork for the complaint."

At this point Zack screamed, "You cannot write me up! I am a doctor and my word is law!"

Darla surprised me when she said, "Maybe in India Zack, maybe in India. But this is Michigan, USA." We left the room and as a parting shot Darla turned to Zack and asked, "Now since you have banned Micheal from your room, would you mind telling me who is going to be your assistant when you are doing your kidney cases and your big prostate cases, now that your main assistant has retired?"

Zack looked uncomfortable and said, "He can assist me for those cases but nothing else." Darla laughed and left the room to file the paperwork the on doctor's attitude.

During my time at the hospital I had three more memorable run-ins with Zack. We were doing an orchiectomy (removal of a testicle) on an older gentleman and Zack was in a hurry, which was an awesome sight, considering he was the fastest suturing surgeon I have ever worked with in any hospital. He placed my retractors and told me not to move for any reason. So, we were doing the case and it was nearing the end and as he was suturing after removing the testicle, he told me to hold a piece of tissue with a raytec sponge. With a last cautioning admonishment to not move or let go, he started to suture. I was just holding the tissue and thinking that the case would end soon and I would be going to another room to do a more pleasant case with a far more pleasant doctor. As I was envisioning that situation I felt two sharp stings in the tips of two of my fingers. I looked down and let go of the tissue to find he had driven the suture through the ends of two of my fingers! "Can't you be careful or did you do on purpose?" I asked.

He looked at me and pulled the suture out of my fingers, which hurt. "You contaminated my suture and you moved. I told you not to move. Why did you not listen to me?"

"Why did you suture two of my fingers

together?"

At this point in time he screamed, "You shut up! You are delaying my case and you have contaminated my suture." I was looking at him in a stunned way as he took the suture to the back table and wiped it off with a saline soaked sponge then returned to the patient and continued to suture. By this time my circulator had called in Darla and told her what had happened. I was sent down to the emergency room for blood tests and examination of the wounds. They gave me an antibiotic just in case of infection. As I was leaving they told me I had one more blood test to do.

I asked, "What now? You have taken at least a quart!" They told me it was for workers comp and it was a drug screen to see if I was under the influence of anything when the accident happened. I was shocked and told them they were insulting me and I wanted to see the union rep about this. Well to make a long story short to save the state, the comp company, and the hospital money they drug test you so they can possibly find some way to avoid paying.

I took the test and passed it, of course. As the holder of a nursing license I would do nothing stupid that could cost me my license. Now all I had to do was take my three month and six month blood test to see if I was going to die from AIDS or not.

Six months, to the day, later I took my last blood test and all was fine. Later that afternoon I did an Ambicor procedure with Zack; basically we were inserting a device to allow a man to achieve an erection when he is totally impotent. Zack was a master of these procedures and you had to be fast to keep up. One of his quirks was a love for a long-handled scalpel with a number ten blade. When he was using the knife, he would be occupied for about five minutes as he delicately dissected tissue in the underside of the penis. The time he spent doing the dissection gave the tech time to clean up the surgical field and get the instruments back on the mayo stand. I was starting to do this when I caught movement out of the corner of my eye. Zack was flipping his scalpel back onto the drape. The scalpel flew like an arrow toward my left hand. I jerked my hand back as fast as I could but his flick and the distance the scalpel flew made it impossible for it to miss me. I felt a sharp stinging pain in the middle finger of my left hand and looked down to see approximately a quarter inch of the number ten blade stuck in my finger… in the bone of my finger.

I let out a curse and pulled the blade from my hand. Tossing the scalpel on the mayo stand, I called the nurse over. "Martha, would you please get me another pair of gloves and dump alcohol and then betadine over my finger, since Zack has impaled it?"

She said, "Again? Is he out to get you? Didn't you just finish the tests from the last time he stuck you?"

I grunted, "Yeah, the little shit seems to have a penchant for stabbing and sticking me."

Zack looked up and screamed, "You will not call me a little shit and you have to stop contaminating my instruments and equipment! You are delaying my case. Now give me my blade back!"

I laughed, "You will wait until I am ready, you little shit. It will be a couple of minutes so why don't you just sit down and calm down. Furthermore, I will not give you back that blade, you are just too dangerous. Maybe I will get you a butter knife to use instead."

He immediately ran to the surgery door, and pushing it open, started to yell for Darla to get into room two. Darla came in and he immediately started to blame me for slowing down his surgery and not giving him back his instrument to finish his dissection.

Looking at me Darla asked, "Why is Martha dumping alcohol and betadine on your left hand?"

Looking at her I quipped, "No real reason I mean why would I really care if Zack drove a scalpel a quarter inch into my finger bone? Should I really give this little shit back a knife with my blood on it?"

Darla said, "So sarcasm aside Zack got you again with a sharp object and he is now pissed about your attitude towards him?"

I nodded, "Yup, that would seem to be the situation again."

Darla instructed me, "Go to the ER, you know the drill and I will scrub in and finish this case with Zack." So once more I was off to the ER to have a quart of blood drawn and another drug test to see if I was stoned or drunk. Once again, I wasn't, but I was beginning to think that maybe it was not such a bad idea.

The third and final incident with Zack was different. It didn't involve me getting injured, but it still involved me getting blamed for everything that went wrong. I was scheduled to do a nephrectomy with Zack as his assistant and had to show a new tech the instruments and explain what we would be doing, as he was not familiar with urology surgeries. We started early so I could explain to the tech what the instruments were used for and when.

As we were talking, in walked Zack who immediately shouted, "Shut up! I cannot work with all this noise."

It was one of those times when you just get tired of the BS and you must say something, "Look Zack, I am teaching here, the case has not started yet because the patient is not even in the room, and I would appreciate it if you would just go away, we are busy here." Having said that, I turned back to the other tech and picked up a pedicle clamp, used to clamp off the arteries to the kidney so the bleeding can be controlled. Zack kept mumbling about the disgraceful attitude I had and eventually stomped out of the room.

A few minutes later I was finished teaching and the patient arrived for the surgery. In walked Zack, scrubbed and ready to be gowned and gloved. The new tech took care of that, not saying a word in the process, and I started to drape the patient for surgery. Again, not a sound, no talking, we were just doing our jobs.

We started the case and the new tech was handling the case just fine; it was nice to have someone listen to instructions and follow them. The only sound was when Zack called for an instrument followed by the sound of it being slapped into his hand. We had the kidney isolated and ready to be removed, and because it was the way Zack likes to do things we were freeing the ureter up so he could send the whole specimen, kidney and ureter, to pathology. I never understood why he did that, but that was Zack.

As we were working I noticed Zack's hands start to shake and he began fumbling with the instrument. I looked up at his face just in time to see his eyes roll back and he went rigid. He started to fall backwards and I reached across the table and grabbed him by the gown, holding him up while the new tech ran around behind him to support him to the floor. At this point all hell broke loose as the nurse hit the panic button that calls a Code Blue. The new tech changed his gloves and we covered the surgical site with towels and moved our back table away from the excitement that was building. We had five doctors, three anesthesia providers, a handful of nurses, and random administration types in the room.

We protected our field, the patient, and generally told people to get the hell out of the room if they were not doing anything besides rubber necking. About five minutes into the panic Zack opened his eyes and shouted at me, "This is all your fault! You would not shut up during the surgery! It's your fault! They put him on a gurney and prepared to take him to the Emergency Room for treatment. He looked up one last time and yelled, "It's your fault! You caused this! I will have you punished!"

As we were wondering who was going to finish the case in walked our worst nightmare - the other urologist on staff and he was a lousy surgeon - slow, sloppy, and arrogant. The case lasted another three hours as he tried to redo everything that was done, using the excuse it was sloppy and not perfect so he would do it. We just rolled our eyes and prayed for time to pass, which it eventually did. The next day we found out that Zack had been self-medicating for a blood pressure problem he had. In the process, he over medicated himself to the point that he literally had no blood pressure when he was standing. He came back to work a week later and taking the properly prescribed medications, his first words were, "It is all your fault. You caused this with all the talking during the case."

I replied, "Talking my ass! You were the only one speaking and you should say thank you that we grabbed your skinny ass and kept you from cracking your skull open on the floor!"

He snorted and stomped off yelling, "You will never be in my room again!"

I smiled to myself and said, "Thank you Jesus." Unfortunately, I was still assigned to his room and we still did cases together but he was mellower, or so it seemed, and I was not injured again...; thank God.

As I mentioned earlier we had another doctor from India working at the hospital as a general surgeon; he hated Zack and the feeling was mutual. Zack would do things to make the other doctor upset, such as eating a beef hamburger in his presence in the locker room or the break room. Bob, the other surgeon, was a strict Hindu and eating beef was, (OMG!) a crime against nature. So, the battles went on between the two of them.

I had the unfortunate, or somewhat dubious, honor to work with Bob because others really didn't like to work with him. Damned seniority got me there. Bob was a general surgeon who thought that there was nothing he could not do, if given a flier to read up on it and a victim, I mean patient, to try it on. Bob was once given a dinner by the hospital for the great accomplishment of getting the surgical time for his Triple A surgeries down to ten hours from the previous fourteen hours. He thought they were honoring him, when they were actually being cynical as normal surgeons took roughly three hours to do a similar case.

At the time, I was employed at the hospital I became the tech for all Bob's Triple A's, not an honor I would seek nor wish on anyone, even my worst enemy, and you would shudder to know some of the things I have wished on my worst enemy. When Bob first started out doing these surgeries he would have other surgeons helping him as assistants. It eventually became one surgeon helping and that was a gyn doctor who was bored. He finally refused to help any further after a particularly bad case on a weekend. This left, horror of horrors, the tech to be his first assistant, another tech to be the primary scrub, and a third tech to be the second scrub. However, as most of these cases happened on weekends or during call, we all learned to check the caller ID before answering the phone if we were not on call. If the ID showed up as the hospital, we would unplug the phones or turn them off and shudder, thinking, *OMG, is it another Bob case?!?*

If the case fell during regular hours we were of course screwed and stuck for the duration. I, for some reason, was always the first assistant with two of my colleagues being the scrubs. Anesthesia was extremely unhappy with the cases because Bob was always ordering something to be hung and infused. It was not uncommon to use ten or more bags of platelets, thirty liters of IV fluid, five to ten units of blood, and God knows how much plasma.

A pattern started to emerge in the cases and I thought that it seemed strange no one else noticed what was happening. Well, I thought no one else noticed. We would be doing the surgery and Bob would be giving random orders to the anesthesia people. I would be cauterizing and clamping bleeders while he made his way down to the aorta. He would find the aorta and then we would heparinize the patient to cut down on the formation of clots while we clamped off the aorta, so we could repair the aneurysm. Waiting patiently with aortic clamp in hand, I listened for Bob to say, "Here clamp it here, no not there, here." It didn't matter that he was guiding the business end of the clamp, it was my fault for the initial faulty placement, which happened every time we did the surgery. The interesting part was he ended up clamping where the initial, "no not here, but here" occurred.

We were now dissecting the artery so we could remove clot and plaque and then trim up the ends of the artery so we could attach the vascular graft. It was then that we would have most of our blood loss, since Bob would open the clamp to flush out bad vapors or evil creatures or something. Granted, we needed to soak the graft in some blood to clot it, which would keep it from leaking through the walls of the graft. However, Bob always seemed amazed at how much blood could come from the aorta, as he would stand and watch for a few seconds as I was holding two suctions for the cell saver in the wound to save what blood we could. Eventually, he would clamp the artery and throw the graft into the abdomen to languish in the blood that was still pooled in the wound. I would stop suctioning while he clotted the graft and then remove the remaining blood. Somewhere along the line, we would lose a good amount of blood and since anesthesia was always checking the labs and giving Bob the results, he would order blood, platelets, plasma, or whatever else he deemed necessary for the case.

Now as surgery progressed it became apparent that things were not going well, and on several occasions, I looked up and saw that the anesthesia people were turning things off. This occurred during several cases around the six-hour mark. Bob would be attaching the graft to the aorta and suturing it in place, when anesthesia would announce that the patient had died and there was nothing that could be done, so it was time to close up. Bob would mumble, "Don't bother me right now, I am doing delicate work and can't be disturbed." Anesthesia would just roll their eyes and continue to shut down their machines, disconnecting cables and monitors from the patient. Bob was oblivious and continued to suture. We would get some big stitches, called bolsters, so that he could do a rapid closure when Bob would finally realize that the patient had passed. Now don't get me wrong, we had cases where the patients survived and did very well, so maybe it was just the quality of patient that Bob had and not him… NAH!

Bob had a fascination with new technology and spared no expense (hospital expense that is) in obtaining it. He would attend a seminar or a workshop over a weekend and come back the master of whatever they talked about and demonstrated. He would bring the brochures and catalogs to the board meetings and pitch his cause as to why he needed the equipment and how much money it would bring in for the hospital. He normally forgot to mention the overall expense of buying it however, and the board just rubber stamped what he wanted. (I told you the hospital was poorly run.)

He wanted a new system for performing vein stripping. At the time, there was a procedure we called the "Death of a Thousand Cuts" which involved many small incisions in the patient's leg, so we could strip out the vein that was varicose. There was another procedure which he didn't like, due to the lack of surgery involved. In the other procedure, the doctor would inject a chemical that caused the vein to scar and occlude. No surgery meant no fun for Bob. Now he had a new procedure he could advertise and perform. It was simple, all he had to do was make two incisions in the patient's leg, use the endoscopic equipment, and basically be done. Bob was really enthused with the equipment however, he also didn't trust the new equipment fully, so he proceeded to do the regular surgery on the patient after using the very expensive endoscopic equipment. The administration never figured out what Bob did. All we knew was that that Bob had found a way to charge more and make the surgery last an hour longer.

At one time, he convinced the administration he needed a laser for his surgeries. We all cringed at the thought of Bob with a laser. He got the laser and seemed to take a real interest in the operation of it. We were impressed until the first time we did surgery with Bob and his new toy. He somehow managed to set the drapes on fire and to burn not one, but two employees. One night shortly after that the laser had an accident that somehow misaligned and broke a couple of mirrors in the system. It went off to be repaired and somehow never returned. Strangely enough, Bob didn't say anything about its leaving, probably at the advice of his lawyer, as two people and a patient were asking for money from someone for their injuries.

Before leaving the chronicles of Bob I will say that we messed with him on every occasion we could. We would glue his OR shoes to the ceiling of the men's locker room. We would glue his locker shut or change the lock with one that looked the same. He really didn't seem to understand that we were messing with him though. Guess he figured that his shoes just got bored and glued themselves to the ceiling. Maybe he thought he had brought the wrong keys for his lock, even if he had used the right key just an hour before.

Finally, there was the Prince of Darkness, or as we called him the POD. This man was the nastiest, meanest, and most disagreeable human being I have ever had the misfortune to work with during surgery. Outside the hospital he was a different creature but inside the doors he was the hell spawn of Satan. The POD made life miserable for everyone who worked with him.

I once asked Darla if it would do any good to file a complaint against the POD?

She laughed and said, "Come with me." We headed down to administration where she showed me a file of complaints against him. I swear they would make a stack three feet high if they were an inch. Darla then turned to me with a smile and asked, "So you think another complaint will solve the problem? He has taken a half dozen anger management classes and caused two of the instructors to quit in anger." She then laughed and said, "So just find a way to deal with him short of murder or maiming."

My first meeting with the POD went none too smoothly. I was an extra tech during a case, and was supposed to observe the procedure to see how it was done at this hospital. More of a learning, not participating experience. So, while the crew was assisting the doctor with draping, I was watching and learning his preferences and quirks. After the draping was finished, I waited for the procedure to start in earnest.

The POD turned towards me and in a sarcastic, yet syrupy, voice said, "Hopkins get your lazy ass over here we have no observers in this room." He stood looking at me as if waiting for me to say something, or to apologize. I just looked at him raised my right hand and extended my middle finger. I then walked up to take my place, even though none was available. He continued to look at me and in a low voice said, "Did you just flip me off?"

To which I replied, "You are pretty observant aren't you, Doctor? Guess I can't get anything past you."

He snorted and said, "I believe you are a smart ass and I don't like smart asses."

I told him, "It's okay, you will probably be kicking me out of your room and we won't have to worry about a friendship anyway." We both turned to the sound of someone trying to not laugh, and doing a poor job of it. The anesthesia provider was red in the face and shaking with laughter that he could not subdue.

The POD looked and said in a voice that would have frozen the sun, "Just what have you found that would cause you to exhibit such jocularity?"

Anesthesia replied between chuckles, "I see two alpha males, one old and skilled and one young and fearless; should be an interesting time in surgery with you two."

To which the POD said, "We will see, we will see." This seemed to set the scene with us, him being domineering and me being resistant to his game. We fought with words and actions, trying to make the other uncomfortable.

I must admit sometimes it was fun to be with the POD when it was someone else who set him off. One night we were called in at 3 a.m. for a fractured hip in the Emergency Room. When we got there the POD looked at the x-rays and shouted out one of his favorite expletives, then turned to me and said, "Find the fracture, Hopkins."

I looked at the x-rays and all I could see was a hip prosthesis which was in place, and the only thing that looked like a fracture was where the femur had been plated and wired during the total joint surgery. The new hip was about a month post-op and the fracture was healing fine. I said, "I remember the case. The femur cracked when we put in the prosthesis and we plated, screwed, and wired the bone. Is that what you wanted me to see?"

The POD nodded and said, "Come with me, we have someone to talk to." Off we went and eventually found the ER doctor. "Would you kindly show me the fracture you got my crew and myself out of bed to come and take care of?"

The ER doctor looked taken aback, but pointed at the fracture with the plate, screws, and wires. He stated in a 'I know more then you' voice. It's right here, about fifteen centimeters down from the proximal end of the femur."

The POD said, "You are pretty damned observant, but seriously you are an idiot. You saw an old fracture which has been reduced and repaired with hardware and you called me and my crew in to fix something that has already been fixed."

The ER doc started to make rumbling sounds about how he was a professional and would not be spoken to that way, when the POD pushed him up against the wall and said, "Come on, Mr. Professional, let's settle our differences in the back parking lot."

The ER doc lost all his color and made a dash from the room vowing to call the hospital CEO first thing in the morning.

The POD said, "Make the phone call about nine or so. That's when he and I have breakfast together at the local Denny's."

To make a long story short the ER doc didn't return to the hospital after Sunday breakfast.

The POD enjoyed making people feel small and ignorant. It seemed to be his mission in life. I was pretty much immune to his actions, having come from a family of fourteen brothers and sisters, you learned to survive or they would eat you up. We butted heads on numerous occasions, it seemed to be a game we both enjoyed. I tried for six years to get thrown out of his room, banned, denied access. I failed miserably, he just wouldn't do it. He would make a statement during surgery to some obscure reference in science or literature and as the others looked at him blankly, I would generally have a comeback. Not because I am brilliant, but because I am very well read. I used to read five books a week for relaxation, any kind of book: science, politics, religion, or history, it didn't matter and this gave me some advantage with the POD.

There was one occasion when the stars and planets were in proper alignment that I could mess with the POD for an entire case. It also allowed me to make the nurse, who absolutely worshiped and feared the POD, just a little crazier than she was already. We were doing a repair of an ACL (Anterior Cruciate Ligament) on a rather large patient. The knee was larger than my head and the joint was protected by very thick layers of fat. Visualization was not easy even though we were trying to do the case arthroscopically, eventually we had to open the knee to do the surgery old school.

We were three hours into an hour and a half surgery. Nothing was going the way it should. We took a patellar graft, to replace the ruptured ligament. Having drilled and prepared the site to accept the graft, the POD took it off my back table and as he prepared to start the insertion, the graft slipped from his fingers, fell to his lap and slithered onto the floor. The air became blue with cursing. The POD was pissed, upset, and looking for someone to blame for his accident.

He looked over at me and I said, "Don't even think about it. I never touched your graft, you and only you, handle grafts; your own policy." He just glared and continued to curse.

Our nurse ran over, pale as a ghost, and suggested, "Doctor I could get you some alcohol and betadine to clean off the graft. Shall I go and get it.

The POD stopped cursing and turned to glare at the nurse. In the softest voice I had heard since my time in the service he hissed, "Now that is just a damned fine idea. I missed out on the five second rule because I was too shocked that I dropped it. Now you come and suggest to me that we take and pick up the graft from the floor, place it in alcohol and then betadine, and implant it in this patient's huge assed knee. Are you stupid, or are you trying to get me sued, and maybe cause this patient a life-threatening infection? I thought you went to nursing school and learned something about asepsis and sterile technique. You did go to nursing school I assume, because if not, you would be doing something else with your life rather than making totally asinine suggestions to me."

The nurse turned even paler and stuttered, "I went to nursing school and I learned about asepsis and sterility but I just thought…"

At this point the POD interrupted her and shouted, "You did not think! You are incapable of thought! You are only good to fill space in my room and breathe the air I breathe!"

Tears welled up in the nurse's eyes and she turned away, only to hear the POD demand, "Run your skinny ass down to the lab and get me a donor graft from the freezer and don't waste any time! GO NOW! GO! Why are you still here?"

The next sound heard in the room was running feet and a door closing. The nurse was on her way to the lab. Now there was a procedure in our lab for removing implantable items and taking them to surgery. You had to have an order from the doctor, you had to have the patient information to enter the implant book, and you had to pray there was an allograft in the freezer for the purpose you needed it for. Our nurse arrived without a doctor's order, she didn't have the patient information, but she lucked out, there was an allograft that would work for our surgery. She came back to the room and the POD looked up at her and sweetly asked, "Where is my graft? Are you hiding it on your person or did you lose it somewhere? I don't see the graft."

Our nurse stuttered, "Doctor, I need, um I

need…"

"What you damned well need is to stop screwing around and get the graft open on the table so I can prepare it for implant. That my dear, is what you need."

She answered, "No, I need an order from you for the lab to give me the graft."

The POD turned beet red and screamed, "Dial the lab and do it now!" She did this and when the lab answered, the POD yelled across the room, "This is Doctor (name withheld to keep from being sued), I need an allograft for my patient and I need it now, so give it to my nurse without any further BS on your part, and let me finish my surgery! Hang up the phone nurse!"

Our nurse grabbed the patient's information and was off to the lab to retrieve the required allograft. Ten minutes later she returned with it in her hand. Entering the room, she waved it like a captured battle flag and exclaimed, "I have it, Doctor, I have it right here." She continued to wave it around.

The POD looked at her and snarled, "Stop with the damned waving and chattering. Give the graft to me and then go sit down, shut your mouth and be a good, quiet little nurse."

The graft was opened on the back table and our furious surgeon took the frozen graft, placing it in warm saline to thaw and become manageable. After a few minutes, he could measure and size the graft to the size needed for the procedure. He turned to the patient, rechecked the site, and being satisfied, turned back to get the graft. I was holding a large basin about the size of a dishpan in my hands with the graft in the middle of the bottom on a moist sponge. "What the hell are you doing, Hopkins? You don't touch my grafts, you know that."

I snickered and replied, "Well, Doctor, we don't want to have lightning strike twice with a graft, do we? I figured if you were to suffer from a déjà vu moment and drop yet another graft it would probably kill our nurse, and I don't want to be an accomplice in that."

He just grabbed the graft with both hands and started putting it in place. The next fifteen minutes went off without a hitch and the graft was in place and secured. It was ready to do its job. We were starting to close the wound when I decided it was time to mess with the POD. The other tech had been sitting quietly during the whole procedure, not saying a word. The POD held out his hand for the next suture and I held it in my left hand, in my right hand I held the local injection we used at the end of the case, this I handed to the doctor. He took it, then stopped to look at it, and to look at me, with a confused look on his face. The nurse, seeing the POD had a local in his hand, ran over and shut off the video equipment and unplugged the camera and light source. The POD was still holding the syringe and I reached over, took it, and gave him the suture he needed to start the closure. He grabbed the scope and camera to take one last look inside at his handy work, but there was nothing on the screen. "Who the hell shut off my video equipment?" he barked.

The nurse said, "I did, you are using a local so we are done with it."

"Get your skinny ass over here and hook me

back up! I am not done and I will tell you when I am."

The nurse scrambled over to hook everything up and turn it back on. The other tech and I were watching her do this and saw she made a mistake but declined to let her know about it. The POD turned his back on her and was looking at the monitor. When the picture came up he started to look around but everything went black on the screen. The POD demanded, "Nurse, fix the damned video. You know how to turn it on and hook it up, don't you?"

Our nurse rushed over to start it up and made the same mistake again. The POD started to look and POOF the screen went black again. The nurse looked devastated and rushed to restart everything, under the glaring eyes of the POD. Again, the same mistake and now the doctor was furious, while the other tech was holding back the laughter tears rolling down his face; I was in a similar situation. I took pity on the nurse and told her, "You are pushing the play button, not the record button; it plays back the last six seconds and then there is nothing, that is why the screen is black. Just push record." The POD turned to me, glaring but didn't say a word. The video remained on and he made his final inspection and held his hand out for the suture. I again handed him the syringe of local and the nurse made a beeline to unplug everything.

The POD glared at me, and screamed at the nurse, "Get the hell away from my equipment! Leave it alone, don't touch it, don't breathe on it, don't even look at it! Sit down, and stay sitting down until I tell you to do something. Do I Make Myself Clear?" Our nurse nodded and rushed back to her chair. The POD turned to me and demanded, "Why the hell are you giving me that damned syringe of local? I use it at the end and you damned well know I use it then! What are you doing?"

I said in a very clear, pouty voice, "I am sick of this case, I am sick of you, and I just want the surgery to be over so I can have a cigarette and try to blank you from my mind." The other tech finally lost it and started to laugh. The nurse turned pale as a ghost and tried to make herself invisible, and anesthesia just snickered.

The case continued and eventually he took the local, which I offered at every opportunity. He wanted to give me a lecture on respect and obedience. I was tired, not in the mood, and just wanted to mess with him for the way he had picked on the nurse.

I said he was a different person outside of the hospital, and he was. He was my orthopedic doctor and my wife's when she had a motor cycle accident. He paid for a well for a tech whose husband was recovering from extensive cancer surgery, and he paid off the home of a tech in our department, who was dying of cancer. He was a study in contrasts. Every Christmas he would walk up to me while I was scrubbing in for a case and put two hundred dollars in my scrub top pocket. He would walk off and say, "Don't you dare thank me. It's for your wife and new grandkids." He was a strange duck to be sure.

We eventually came to a truce after causing each other minor injuries and inconveniences. I think the turning point came during a total knee we were doing. The POD was driving the trial into place when he cursed and the mallet flew from his hand and landed on the floor. He was cursing up a blue streak and I noticed the thumb on his right hand had dislocated. I reached over, took his hand in my right hand, and pulled his thumb back in to place with my left hand. He just looked at me and called for another mallet. The new mallet was opened and he started to finish his placement. His thumb dislocated again. I put it back in place; luckily this time the mallet fell on the field. He picked it up again and I took it from his hand, handed him the impactor, and hammered the trial into place. He didn't say anything and the case continued.

When everything was ready, we opened the components for the knee. After placing the femoral component where he wanted it, he took the mallet, looked at it, then handed it to me. I pounded the prosthesis into place. He held out his hand and took the mallet in his other hand and tapped the impactor, then handed the mallet back. We placed the remaining components in much the same way. The ones that needed to be put in place with a mallet I pounded into position and he put on a final tap. This became the way we did total joints for the next four years.

My wife and I would still be at that hospital if it didn't fall under a new administration, who tried to circumvent the union and take away benefits. I just didn't want the fight. So, we decided it was time to take up jobs as traveling nurses and get paid while seeing the country.

I had some wild times with people as a traveler, but that is another story for a later time. On my last day, they had a going away party for me, which I thought was very nice. The POD came and shook my hand and told me as much of an asshole as I was, he would miss me in his room. He then handed me a box with a bottle of twenty-five-year-old Single Malt Scotch inside. I was touched, as this was a great Scotch.

We left the next day and have not been back to Michigan since. I heard the POD was in an accident coming home from a hunting trip and flipped his Humvee on black ice. He broke both shoulders and it ended his career. It was really too bad, because despite his demeanor, he was a brilliant surgeon. I hope he is doing well.

My wife Carol and I traveled across the country, from coast to coast learning about places we had never been and doing things that just sounded fun. Carol had her first train ride ever in New York.

If the truth were to be told, working as a traveler exposed me to more of the bizarre that the medical field had to offer. More often than not it was the people that were strange this time, not the hospital and not the surgeons, well not all the surgeons. But that is another book for another time.

About the Author

Micheal is a Vietnam Veteran. After leaving the Army, he joined the Air Force to learn some sort of useful career. Being a Combat Medic and Demolitions Specialist really didn't have a lot of salability in the Post-Vietnam era. He could have been a mercenary, but his wife put her foot down firmly on that thought. So, he joined the Air Force to learn a trade. After testing, he was told he qualified for every enlisted job the Air Force had to offer but he was not qualified to be a clerk. He turned down Crypto, Air Traffic Control, Language School, and Computers. Not being the brightest firefly on the river, Micheal thought that computers would not be a big thing. So, he chose Operating Room Technician and has not regretted one minute of his career. It has paid the bills for years and given him great pleasure to work with the people in surgery. It also gave him the basis of this book.

Poetry by Micheal Hopkins is also available.

Visit http://www.shywindcreations.com

Made in the USA
Monee, IL
14 September 2026

62974513R00095